Teleneurology

Edited by Richard Wootton and Victor Patterson

Teleneurology

Edited by

Richard Wootton

Centre for Online Health, University of Queensland, Brisbane, Australia

Victor Patterson

Royal Victoria Hospital, Belfast, UK

Foreword by

Charles Warlow

Professor of Medical Neurology, University of Edinburgh, Edinburgh, UK

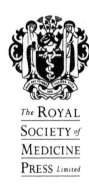

The ROYAL
SOCIETY *of*
MEDICINE
PRESS *Limited*

British Library Cataloguing in Publication Data
A catalogue record for this book is available from the British Library.

ISBN 1-85315-671-X

Distribution in Europe and Rest of World:
Marston Book Services Ltd
PO Box 269
Abingdon
Oxon OX14 4YN, UK
Tel: +44 (0)1235 465500
Fax: +44 (0)1235 465555
Email: direct.order@marston.co.uk

Distribution in the USA and Canada:
Royal Society of Medicine Press Ltd
c/o Jamco Distribution Inc
1401 Lakeway Drive
Lewisville, TX 75057, USA
Tel: +1 800 538 1287
Fax: +1 972 353 1303
Email: jamco@majors.com

Distribution in Australia and New Zealand:
Elsevier Australia
30–52 Smidmore Street
Marrickville, NSW 2204
Australia
Tel: + 61 2 9517 8999
Fax: + 61 2 9517 2249
Email: service@elsevier.com.au

Typeset by Phoenix Photosetting, Chatham, Kent
Printed in Great Britain by Bell & Bain Ltd, Glasgow

▶ Contents

▶ List of Contributors

Rustam Al-Shahi Division of Clinical Neurosciences, School of Molecular and Clinical Medicine, University of Edinburgh, Western General Hospital, Edinburgh, UK

Liam Caffery Department of Medical Imaging, Royal Brisbane and Women's Hospital, Herston, Queensland, Australia

Sean Connolly Department of Clinical Neurophysiology, St Vincent's University Hospital, Dublin, Ireland

Alan Coulthard Department of Medical Imaging, Royal Brisbane and Women's Hospital, Herston, Queensland, Australia

John Craig Department of Neurology, Royal Victoria Hospital, Belfast, UK

Mary Fitzsimons Department of Neurophysics, Beaumont Hospital, Dublin, Ireland

Sinead Gormley Outpatient Department, Tyrone County Hospital, Omagh, UK

Jeanette C Hartshorn Telehealth Center, Department of Neurology, School of Nursing, University of Texas Medical Branch, Galveston, Texas, USA

Elsie Hui Medical and Geriatric Unit, Shatin Hospital, Hong Kong, China; Department of Medicine and Therapeutics, The Chinese University of Hong Kong, Hong Kong, China

Mostafa Kamal Centre for the Rehabilitation of the Paralysed, Dhaka, Bangladesh

AJ Larner Department of Neurology, Walton Centre for Neurology and Neuro-surgery, Liverpool, UK

Danny McArdle Department of Teleneurology, Royal Victoria Hospital, Belfast, UK

John McConville Department of Neurology, Royal Victoria Hospital, Belfast, UK

Victor Patterson Department of Neurology, Royal Victoria Hospital, Belfast, UK; Centre for Online Health, University of Queensland, Brisbane, Queensland, Australia

James T Pelekanos Department of Paediatrics and Child Health, Royal Children's Hospital, University of Queensland, Brisbane, Queensland, Australia

Karen A Rasmusson Department of Neurology, School of Nursing, University of Texas Medical Branch, Galveston, Texas, USA

Stephen Read Department of Neurology, Royal Brisbane and Women's Hospital, Herston, Queensland, Australia

Eric S Rosenthal Department of Neurology, Massachusetts General Hospital, Boston, Massachusetts, USA

Lee H Schwamm Department of Neurology, Massachusetts General Hospital, Boston, Massachusetts, USA

Anthony C Smith Centre for Online Health, University of Queensland, Brisbane, Queensland, Australia

Richard Wootton Centre for Online Health, University of Queensland, Brisbane, Queensland, Australia

▶ Foreword

Living and working in Scotland, I am very familiar with the politician's imperative of providing decent healthcare to 'remote and rural communities', even if neurology is not particularly high on their wish list. However, Scottish 'remote and rural' pales into insignificance compared with most parts of the world, certainly with respect to the number and distribution of neurologists who, after all, are the best-placed doctors to deal effectively and efficiently with patients who have a disorder of the nervous system. But what to do to help these patients, many of whom cannot afford specialist care anyway, when there is no neurologist for hundreds or possibly thousands of miles? Although getting the diagnosis right is important, this really matters only if it leads to effective interventions, which, these days, we have in neurology — antiepileptic drugs, antiparkinsonian drugs, drugs for migraine and secondary stroke prevention, and treatment for rarities such as myasthenia gravis. These drugs are not necessarily very expensive if doctors can avoid being bamboozled by the marketing departments of the pharmaceutical industry or if they are prepared to use a cheaper alternative when the much more expensive version is not significantly better or simply is unavailable. It really should make a difference getting a specialized neurological opinion, wherever the patient happens to be.

So, welcome teleneurology, the neurological branch of telemedicine that allows specialist neurologists to communicate with less specialized colleagues and their patients, whether they be just down the road, on a remote island in the same country, up in the air, or in a completely different country. As long as they can speak or read the same language, then the telephone, email and videoconferencing can bring them together to discuss individual cases or more general issues of importance. In the old days, consultant neurologists from London used to cover most of the south of England by motoring down to the distant city, doing a clinic, having a nice dinner in a congenial hotel, and motoring back the next day – once a month, or even less often. Teleneurology will do, and is doing, better than this in those parts of the world where there is still poor access to neurologists. Of course, it could do even better, and this book should help.

Teleneurology is one of a series of books on telemedicine. It has been put together by – appropriately – a neurologist who practises teleneurology and an expert on telemedicine in general. They have arranged the book to describe the techniques available, how to use these techniques effectively, and the applications to some common neurological problems. I hope it does well. It would be comforting to think that if I should fall neurologically sick in some remote corner of the world, then it would have available email or a simple telephone, if not a videoconferencing studio, through which my doctor could obtain the best possible neurological advice.

Charles Warlow
Professor of Medical Neurology, University of Edinburgh
Edinburgh, UK

▶ Preface

This is the sixth book in the Royal Society of Medicine's telemedicine series, a series of multi-author books on telemedicine topics designed to provide examples of best practice in their respective fields. Its predecessors are:

- *The Legal and Ethical Aspects of Telemedicine*, BA Stanberry, 1998
- *Introduction to Telemedicine*, R Wootton and J Craig (eds), 1999
- *Teledermatology*, R Wootton and A Oakley (eds), 2002
- *Telepsychiatry and e-Mental Health*, R Wootton, P Yellowlees and P McLaren (eds), 2003
- *Telepediatrics: Telemedicine and Child Health*, R Wootton and J Batch (eds), 2005.

This book describes how telemedicine can be applied to neurology. Teleneurology is practised around the world, and the book's contributors, who come from six countries on four continents, reflect this. All have practical experience, the majority are practising clinicians, and most have published in detail on their respective subjects. This book presents the experience of practitioners across a wide range of applications of telemedicine in neurology.

The idea for this book was conceived some years ago at a stage when the subject was in its infancy; the discipline has now matured to some extent. A six-month sabbatical at the Centre for Online Health for one of the editors (VP) made its realization possible. It is a pleasure to acknowledge the contribution of Questmark, a prominent UK supplier of videoconferencing systems and services, towards the costs of producing the book. In this, they have been supported by Tandberg, to whom we are also grateful.

The aim of the book is to show how telemedicine can be applied to neurology and to challenge clinicians to consider it in their everyday working practice. Although it is most relevant to practising neurologists, many chapters will also be of interest to health service managers, planners and information technology staff. We think that anyone involved in telemedicine will find the material interesting, because much of it is relevant to other fields as well as neurology.

This book is divided into three sections:

- techniques
- applications
- practical issues.

The emphasis is on the utility of the technique rather than the technology itself. We have therefore deliberately kept the technical information to a minimum. Readers who are anxious for more may consult previous books in the series. We hope that within the broad spectrum of ideas expressed within this book, everyone will find something of relevance to their individual practice. We hope you enjoy reading it.

Richard Wootton and Victor Patterson
Centre for Online Health, University of Queensland
Brisbane, Queensland, Australia

Section 1: Techniques

1. **Introduction**
   Victor Patterson and Richard Wootton

2. **Teleneurology by Telephone**
   AJ Larner

3. **Teleneurology by Email**
   Victor Patterson

4. **Teleneurology by Videoconferencing**
   John Craig

▶1

Introduction

Victor Patterson and Richard Wootton

Introduction

Neurological diseases are common the world over. Stroke is a major cause of death and disability globally, epilepsy affects more than 1% of the world's population, and motor-vehicle accidents with subsequent brain injury causing major disability are a true pandemic, particularly in young men. Neurologists – the doctors with specialized expertise and training in neurological disease – can make a difference to many patients with these diseases. Unfortunately, the distribution of neurologists throughout the world is patchy: in New York there is a neurologist for approximately every 20 000 people, whereas in Myanmar the Mandalay region has a neurologist for every 2.5 million people. Some countries have no specialized neurologists at all.[1] Even in highly industrialized countries such as the USA, there can be very limited access to neurologists in rural areas because of the tendency of neurologists to practise in urban centres.

Training more neurologists may seem the obvious answer to this mismatch between demand and supply, but it may not solve the problem for a number of reasons. First, doctors from developing countries, who have to go to the industrialized world for postgraduate training, often stay in the industrialized world instead of returning home. Second, if such doctors do return to their own countries, they are more likely to work in private practice, so many people may be unable to afford their services. Third, these doctors are more likely to practise in large cities, so the rural population may be unable to reach them.

Teleneurology

So, can teleneurology help? Telemedicine is the practice of medicine using modern communication technologies when the doctor and the patient are separated in place and possibly in time. The modern communication technologies involved are nothing more alarming or threatening than the telephone, email and videoconferencing. Telemedicine has been applied successfully to other specialties, particularly radiology and psychiatry, but neurology has been a slow starter. In a recent survey of US telemedicine programmes, neurology activity was fifth in terms of frequency of use by those programmes that reported their activities, coming after mental health, paediatrics, cardiology and dermatology.[2] Indeed, as a specialty, neurology may be very suitable for this type of medicine. Neurology is an auditory and visual rather than tactile subject – the skill is in recognizing diseases principally from a history, backed up by demonstrating physical signs in an examination. A history can be obtained directly in a videolink or by proxy in an email message or telephone call from another doctor. An examination can be either witnessed by videolink or taken on trust from another doctor when email is used. So, if neurologists based in urban centres can deal with neurological patients in distant parts of the country, or even different countries, by means of communication technology, then the problem of reduced access to specialist care will be lessened, if not solved.

Telemedicine of a sort is already part of the daily practice of most neurologists. One example is meeting a colleague, either professionally or socially, who describes a case and asks for an opinion. Another example is a colleague, or indeed a patient, telephoning and asking for advice. In both of these everyday situations, the neurologist and the colleague or the patient clearly are not in the same place, and advice on diagnosis and management may be given without seeing the patient. Whether or not it is necessary for the patient to be seen and examined personally depends on the clinical judgement of the neurologist, and it is this use of clinical judgement that pervades every other aspect of teleneurology. Ultimately, if a face-to-face examination is necessary to sort out a problem, then such an examination needs to be done.

Another important point about teleneurology is that it is not an end in itself, or a quasi-religion; rather, it is merely a possible solution to problems that neurologists have in their everyday practice. The problem addressed earlier of inadequate access to a neurologist in many parts of the world is perhaps the most important problem faced by patients and neurologists alike, but there are many others. These problems may be specific to countries, to healthcare delivery systems or indeed to individual neurologists. Before even considering whether telemedicine might help, the problem needs to be formulated clearly. For example, one problem that is crying out for a telemedicine solution is how to provide neurological input to patients with motor neurone disease and who are too disabled to travel to clinics.

Evaluation

Telemedicine is more likely to be accepted by the neurological community if it is subjected to proper evaluation. Each new telemedicine application within neurology needs to be evaluated in a number of different ways (Table 1.1). Feasibility, acceptability and initial safety are essential hurdles that must be jumped before more detailed evaluation is performed. Although some initial feasibility work can be done in a laboratory setting, the main pilot study needs to be carried out in a practice situation to see whether it works. Acceptability to patients is rarely a problem in any telemedicine application,[3] but it is crucial to the success of any project that the staff members who use it are happy doing so; therefore, this needs to be measured and appropriate modifications made if necessary. A study of initial safety should compare the telemedicine application with the gold standard – usually face-to-face examination. If this initial safety is poor, then the study should be abandoned or its

Table 1.1. Evaluations necessary before implementing a new telemedicine application

Evaluation	Method
Feasibility	Pilot study
Acceptability to patients	Structured questionnaire
Acceptability to staff	Structured questionnaire
Initial safety	Comparison with gold standard
Effectiveness	Clinical or managerial assessment
Cost	Comparison with conventional care
Long-term safety	Long-term follow-up of patients treated
Sustainability	Continuing use after study ends

execution changed. Initial safety is crucial to give clinicians the confidence to proceed in an area where they may feel exposed medicolegally.

Such a study can provide only preliminary judgement on whether a procedure is truly safe. A more reliable estimate will come from longer-term patient follow-up, looking for outcome measures such as death or change in diagnosis – the more patients involved and the longer the follow-up, the better. Interpretation of results may, however, be limited by the paucity of this sort of information for face-to-face examination.

Effectiveness can be judged either clinically – patients diagnosed and managed effectively – or managerially – eg number of treatments delivered within a timeframe. Sometimes, clinical effectiveness can be demonstrated in a single case study, but usually a cohort study is required.

Cost, cost-effectiveness and efficiency studies require costed outcome measures and actions and need a comparison between a telemedicine-treated cohort and a conventionally treated cohort. This is best done prospectively, but it can be performed retrospectively if there is no alternative. Information showing that an application results in cost-savings will help to develop the business case needed to bring it into mainstream service. Even if studies are positive in all of the above findings, the application may still fail to be used after the study, for a number of reasons. Sustainability is the real measure of the success of any telemedicine project.

The design of the necessary studies is not always easy. Single case studies and single cohort studies are easy to perform and can give useful information on feasibility and effectiveness. Such studies are, however, sometimes frowned upon by members of the evidence-based medicine movement. Cohort-comparison studies and randomized controlled trials (RCTs) are more acceptable but often much more difficult to organize in the real-life milieu in which telemedicine is practised. Indeed, in some situations, an RCT may not be possible ethically. We have carried out both of these types of study and had difficulty in each: in an RCT of neurological outpatients, our conventionally managed cohort had the lowest investigation rate of any cohort that we have ever been involved with,[4,5] and in a cohort comparison study, the cohorts were different in age, which was an important confounding variable.[6]

Despite these difficulties, formal evaluations of feasibility, safety, acceptability, effectiveness and cost are important in each application of telemedicine in neurology, just as they should be with any new health-related intervention. This evidence-based approach should ease the passage of teleneurology into neurological practice.

Conclusion

Teleneurology has taken its first hesitant steps towards the mainstream in the past few years, with an increasing trickle of publications documenting its contribution to patient care. A MEDLINE search from 1995 to the present, similar to that used by Youngberry[7] but restricted to neurological headings, illustrates this trend (Fig. 1.1). The purpose of this book is to bring together this published information on teleneurology in a single place and in a form that will stimulate both the use of the technique in everyday clinical practice and the research that is needed to further its progress. Any omissions are the responsibility of the editors.

We hope this book will offer something to all those concerned in delivering neurological services – neurologists, nurses and allied health professionals. The first section deals with the communication techniques that can be used to practise neurology and the evidence supporting their use. The second section provides accounts of the use of teleneurology in both specific neurological conditions and specific applications. In the final section, we have included chapters that we hope will

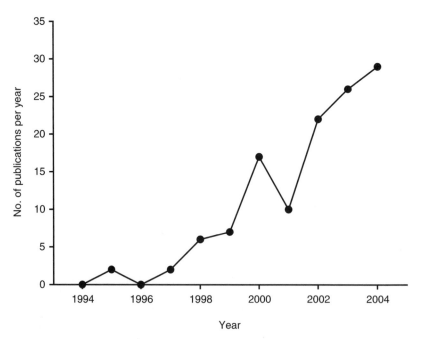

Fig. 1.1. MEDLINE publications on telemedicine and neurological topics from 1995 to 2004. NB: 2004 data are incomplete. Courtesy of K Youngberry.

be of everyday practical use to practitioners in the field. The broad focus of the book is clinical, but we have included technical details where these are important to the understanding of, and use of, the techniques.

We hope you enjoy reading it.

References

1   Bergen DC. Training and distribution of neurologists worldwide. *Journal of Neurological Science* 2002; **198**: 3–7.
2   Grigsby B. *2004 TRC Report on US Telemedicine Activity*. Kingston, NJ: Civic Research Institute, 2004.
3   Mair F, Whitten P. Systematic review of studies of patient satisfaction with telemedicine. *British Medical Journal* 2000; **320**: 1517–1520.
4   Chua R, Craig J, Wootton R, Patterson V. Randomised controlled trial of telemedicine for new neurological outpatient referrals. *Journal of Neurology, Neurosurgery and Psychiatry* 2001; **71**: 63–66.
5   Chua R, Craig J, Esmonde T *et al*. Telemedicine for new neurological outpatients: putting a randomized controlled trial in the context of everyday practice. *Journal of Telemedicine and Telecare* 2002; **8**: 270–273.
6   Craig J, Chua R, Russell C *et al*. A cohort study of early neurological consultation by telemedicine on the care of neurological inpatients. *Journal of Neurology, Neurosurgery and Psychiatry* 2004; **75**: 1031–1035.
7   Youngberry K. Telemedicine research and MEDLINE. *Journal of Telemedicine and Telecare* 2004; **10**: 121–123.

▶2

Teleneurology by Telephone

AJ Larner

Introduction

As the Greek prefix *tele* (τηλε) denotes, telemedicine is medicine from afar, far off or at a distance. Although the word is recent (it does not appear in the second edition of the *Oxford English Dictionary*, published in 1989), the concept is not. From time immemorial, physicians have been consulted by word of mouth or by letter about patients without seeing and examining them, because of the difficulties of travel or the limitations imposed by illness. Indeed, the very practice of writing medical texts, dating from the time of Hippocrates, was prompted, at least in part, by the desire to make medical information and expertise available to those at a distance from the learned author. What has changed in the succeeding centuries is the availability of new technologies for communication over distance, such as the telephone (the subject of this chapter) and, more recently, videoconferencing and the Internet.

Telemedicine by telephone

The telephone has been used to manage demand in health-maintenance organizations[1] and also to provide medical information, advice, outpatient follow-up and triage in a number of medical and surgical specialties. These include paediatrics, pain, oncology, psychiatry, chest medicine, head and neck surgery, diabetes, renal disease and rheumatology. Neurology is conspicuous by its absence from this list.

Nonetheless, there are some examples of telephone telemedicine of particular relevance to neurological practice. The Counselling and Diagnosis in Dementia (CANDID) service was developed by the Dementia Research Group at the National Hospital for Neurology and Neurosurgery in Queen Square, London.[2] In its first two years of operation, over 1000 calls were logged, more than half of which were 'generic', ie emanating from members of the public or health professionals seeking information and advice, rather than from those attending the hospital outpatient clinic. Demand for such services has thus been demonstrated. Telephone interviews in place of face-to-face interviews have been used for the diagnosis of dementia (with cognitive measurement scales adapted for telephone use)[3] and to measure disability in multiple sclerosis.[4] Nurse-led epilepsy clinics supported by a distant neurologist contacted by telephone and, if necessary, videolink have proven feasible and acceptable, if more expensive than face-to-face clinics.[5] Epilepsy nurse specialists can give medication advice as well as information and support by telephone.[6] Epilepsy is also a major component of paediatric neurology, in which specialists are in short supply in many parts of the world. Here, too, a telephone nursing service has been shown to reduce the demand on paediatric neurologists.[7]

Although there are few published articles on telephone teleneurology, it is worth noting that this method of practice is, de facto, the norm in most British district general hospitals. Although about 20% of acute admissions to district general hospitals are for primarily neurological problems, such is the staffing situation and organization of British neurology that few of these patients are actually seen by a neurologist. Reliance therefore is placed, when necessary, on telephone communication with the regional neuroscience centre, calls often being made between a junior hospital doctor and a junior neurologist, a situation that seems to excite no particular comment, far less any audit. Similarly, in a recent textbook on telephone medicine, the chapter on headache contains no references to any formal studies on the use of the telephone in this, the most common neurological symptom.[8]

NHS Direct

NHS Direct is a UK telephone triage service staffed by nurses, giving healthcare advice and information 24 hours a day. It is the largest telemedicine system in the world, dealing with 3.5 million calls in 2001–02,[9] and this is the reason for describing it in some detail here. It was introduced in the UK in 1998 to act as a gateway and reduce attendances at general practitioner (GP) surgeries and hospital accident and emergency (A&E) departments. By the end of 2000, it had been rolled out to the whole of England, Scotland and Wales. Consultations use computer-based assessment support systems, which have defined protocols for specific problems based on clinical algorithms. The average consultation time is 14 minutes.

Early studies found patients to be generally satisfied with information received from NHS Direct,[9,10] but the anticipated effect, a reduced demand for immediate care, was in fact negligible.[11] Indeed, although the service is meant to be complementary to and integrated with other National Health Service (NHS) functions,[1] many GPs and hospital A&E departments dislike NHS Direct, since it refers callers to them ('I rang NHS Direct and they said to go and see my GP/go to A&E').[12,13] Moreover, triage for same-day appointments in general practice by NHS Direct takes longer and is more costly than practice-based triage.[14]

Studies of the diagnostic accuracy of NHS Direct and of the appropriateness of advice given using 'standardized patients' have appeared in both the medical[15] and the lay[16] press, expressing concerns about delayed and incorrect diagnosis. This may simply be a reflection of the tendency of algorithm-based systems of this type to err on the side of making false-positive diagnoses, while false-negative diagnoses may attract adverse and highly public comment (eg a front-page headline in the *Daily Mail* on 14 February 2002 read: 'My Baby Girl was Killed by NHS Direct'). Large differences in outcome have been reported according to the software system being used.[15]

How effective is NHS Direct advice? To date, NHS Direct has not generated any outcome information about its own activities. A study of patients referred to an A&E department by NHS Direct found that about two-thirds followed the advice given.[17] However, there have been concerns that awareness of NHS Direct is low (only 8% of patients questioned directly at an inner-city Teesside general practice in early 2001 were aware of NHS Direct),[18] and use is least among patients whose need for medical advice and information is greatest, such as older people,[19] ethnic minorities, people in low socioeconomic groups and people with established ill health.[20]

NHS Direct and neurology

What influence, if any, does NHS Direct have on neurological practice? Unfortunately, there are no data on NHS Direct calls by specialty. Over the period 2001–04, a number of studies examining whether patients referred to neurology outpatient clinics were aware of and had used NHS Direct were conducted.[21–24] The methodology used has been simple, namely asking consecutive patients referred to general or specialist neurology outpatient clinics whether they were aware of the NHS Direct telephone helpline and, if so, whether they had used it. Although this approach depends on patient recall, and hence may be open to recall bias, it provides some information about the effect of NHS Direct in the context of neurology outpatient clinics.

General neurology clinics

In the initial study, undertaken between January and March 2001 at two district general hospitals in north-west England, shortly after NHS Direct was rolled out in the region, very few (2%) patients had used the service[21]. This changed dramatically within a year.[22]

The data for the January–March cohorts for the years 2002–04 are shown in Figs 2.1 and 2.2. The aggregate data, summing the cohorts from 2002 to 2004, show that out of a total of 656 new patients seen, 348 (53%) had heard of NHS Direct. Of these, 89 (14%, or 26% of those aware of NHS Direct) had used the service. Only three (3%) of these 89 patients volunteered the fact that they had called NHS Direct before being questioned specifically. Of the 89 NHS Direct users, in 27 (30%, or 8% of those aware of NHS Direct, or 4% of the whole cohort), the call was judged to be related to the clinical problem for which they were attending the neurology clinic. Most of the other NHS Direct users were calling on behalf of another family member, usually a child but sometimes an older person.

Fig. 2.2 shows that awareness of NHS Direct was greatest (62%) in the age group 31–40 years but fairly consistent, at more than 50%, from the 21–30 years age group up to and including the 61–70 years age group. Usage was highest (22–25%) in the 21–30 years and 31–40 years age groups, which may reflect, at least in part, the use of the service to enquire about the ailments of young children. These data also confirm a previous report that found elderly people to be less likely to have used NHS Direct.[19]

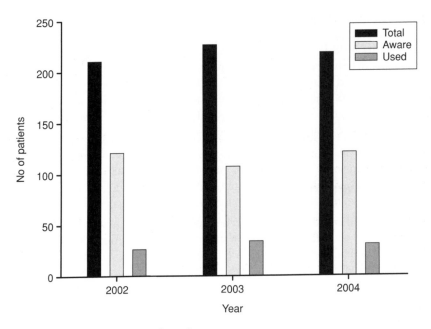

Fig. 2.1. NHS Direct awareness and use, by year.

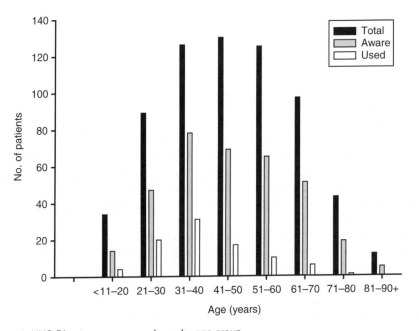

Fig. 2.2. NHS Direct awareness and use, by age group.

Cognitive disorders

A study of NHS Direct awareness and use has also been undertaken in a specialist neurology clinic devoted to the assessment of acquired cognitive problems, predominantly memory disorders, which is based at a regional neuroscience centre with a catchment population in excess of three million people in north-west England and north Wales[23]. Over a six-month period (October 2001–March 2002), there were 104 consultations (73 new patient assessments, 31 follow-up visits). About two-thirds of the patients had cognitive disorders (the majority of these had Alzheimer's disease), while the remainder had psychiatric illness or no objective evidence of cognitive decline. The majority of patients did not attend alone. The result of asking about awareness of NHS Direct was positive in 63 (61%) consultations, higher than might have been anticipated from the age of the patients alone (mean age 62 years; Fig. 2.2; ages of spouses, relatives, friends and carers attending with the patients were not recorded). In 10 cases, NHS Direct had been called (16% of those aware of NHS Direct, 10% of whole cohort), but in only two cases was the call relevant to the reason for referral[23]. Results are summarized in Table 2.1.

Table 2.1. NHS Direct awareness in a cognitive disorder clinic population ($n = 104$) and in a headache population ($n = 208$)

	Population	
	Cognitive disorder clinic	Headache
Total	104	208
Aware	63	120
Used	10	36
Used for presenting problem	2	14

Headache

The most common problem encountered in neurological outpatient practice is headache. The majority of these patients have primary headache disorders and the best management of these problems is still debated. However, a greater role for primary care, as opposed to hospital-based secondary care, has been recommended. In a study of 1000 consecutive new outpatients seen over an approximately 10-month period (2002–03) in general neurology outpatient clinics at two district general hospitals and a regional neuroscience centre, headache was the reason for referral or the principal complaint in the clinic in 208 (21%) patients.[24] Only one patient had a brain tumour, with typical features of raised intracranial pressure (visual obscurations). The remainder had primary headache disorders, mostly tension-type headache (chronic or episodic, $n = 160$) and migraine in its various forms ($n = 34$). Headache patients were asked about their awareness and use of NHS Direct. Of these 208 patients, 120 (58%) had heard of NHS Direct. Of these, 36 (30% of headache patients aware of NHS Direct, 17% of all headache patients) had used the service. Of these 36, the call to NHS

Direct related to headache in 14 (39% of users, 12% of all those aware of NHS Direct, 7% of all headache patients)[24] (see Table 2.1). This percentage is lower than for use of other medical resources by headache patients, such as community pharmacists and the Internet.[25]

The experiences of the 14 headache patients contacting NHS Direct were explored further. Five recollected being told either 'go to hospital' or 'call an ambulance' immediately. The final diagnosis made by the neurologist in these five cases was chronic tension-type headache ($n = 3$), episodic tension type headache ($n = 1$), and migraine without aura ($n = 1$) – the reported NHS Direct diagnosis in this latter case was cerebral haemorrhage. One patient was told to go to a local NHS Walk-in Centre (final diagnosis: chronic tension-type headache), and another two patients were told to attend their GPs (both chronic tension-type headache). NHS Direct diagnosed a transient ischaemic attack in a man subsequently diagnosed by a neurologist as having migraine without headache (migraine equivalent). One patient with chronic tension-type headache was told to lie in a darkened room. One patient phoned for information about side-effects of analgesic medication. Three patients could not recall the outcomes of their calls to NHS Direct. It was concluded that NHS Direct was neither dangerous nor helpful in the management of headache, presumably because algorithms currently in use cannot provide for the taking of an adequate history to inform the advice given.[24] This concurs with another study reporting outcomes dependent on software.[15]

Conclusions

As with all medical interventions, telemedicine by telephone is susceptible to analysis in terms of potential benefits and potential risks. In the specific context of neurological practice, potential benefits are self-evident, such as bringing neurological information and expertise to patients otherwise unable to access them because of distance from neurological centres.[2–5] To reap these potential benefits requires an awareness of the service's existence and a willingness of individual patients to use it in preference to traditional face-to-face consultation. The main risk of computer-based assessment software is incorrect diagnosis, and this itself may promote a tendency to false-positive diagnoses in order to 'be on the safe side'. Furthermore, telephone-based services will not be available to people without a telephone, which may include patients with the greatest medical need, such as elderly people.[19]

Considering NHS Direct, a generic telephone helpline, as a teleneurology service it is questionable whether such a system can deliver clinical benefits without running undue risks. Studies in neurology outpatient clinics suggest that only slightly more than half of the patients attending them are aware of NHS Direct. Moreover, although about one in seven patients aware of NHS Direct has used it, few of these calls relate to the reason for neurological referral. Awareness and use seem to be lower in elderly people. In a discipline where attention to specific historical detail is often of paramount importance in establishing a correct diagnosis, it is doubtful whether computer-based algorithms will be sufficiently well developed to ensure accuracy of neurological diagnosis, reflecting the well-recognized fact that outcome is highly dependent on the software used.[15] Taking as an example headache, the most common reason for neurological referral, advice given by NHS Direct seemed to be neither helpful nor dangerous, with some evidence for false-positive diagnosis of symptomatic headache disorders with ensuing unnecessary use of secondary care resources.[24]

Thus, telephone teleneurology is already here, but the question 'Will telephone teleneurology hit the big time?' remains, in my view, an open one. A tentative answer would acknowledge that the service can be only as good as the algorithms available, just as face-to-face neurology depends on the clinical competence of the practitioner. Just as greater efforts are being made to ensure competency in the training of neurologists, so more effort may be required to develop computer-based algorithms suitable for use with neurological problems. In the meantime, there are other teleneurology resources available to patients, such as Internet websites. With increased home Internet access, patients may prefer these on the grounds that they are more interactive. However, this latter approach has its own difficulties: e-patients sometimes are alarmed unnecessarily by medical information that they have accessed but that is not in fact relevant to their condition, leading to the need for further consultation with doctors, a phenomenon that has been labelled 'cyberchondria'. Teleneurology by telephone might be anticipated to create an analogous problem ('telechondria'). The experience of headache patients calling NHS Direct provides some evidence to support this possibility.[24]

Further information

National Institute of Neurological Disorders and Stroke (NINDS). http://accessible.ninds.nih.gov/index.htm. Accessed 28 January 2005.
Selwa LM, Ozuna J, Taylor L et al. Neuro-Triage Telephone Advice. Boston: Butterworth-Heinemann, 2002.

References

1 Donaldson L. Telephone access to health care: the role of NHS Direct. Journal of the Royal College of Physicians London 2000; 34: 33–35.
2 Harvey R, Roques PK, Fox NC, Rossor MN. CANDID – Counselling and Diagnosis in Dementia: a national telemedicine service supporting the care of younger patients with dementia. International Journal of Geriatric Psychiatry 1998; 13: 381–388.
3 Kawas C, Karagiozis H, Resau L et al. Reliability of the Blessed Telephone Information-Memory-Concentration Test. Journal of Geriatric Psychiatry and Neurology 1995; 8: 238–242.
4 Lechner-Scott J, Kappos L, Hofman M et al. Can the Expanded Disability Status Scale be assessed by telephone? Multiple Sclerosis 2003; 9: 154–159.
5 Bingham E, Patterson V. Nurse-led epilepsy clinics: a telemedicine approach. Journal of Neurology, Neurosurgery and Psychiatry 2002; 73: 216.
6 Hosking PG, Duncan JS, Sander JW. The epilepsy nurse specialist at a tertiary care hospital: improving the interface between primary and tertiary care. Seizure 2002; 11: 494–499.
7 Letourneau MA, MacGregor DL, Dick PT et al. Use of a telephone nursing line in a pediatric neurology clinic: one approach to the shortage of subspecialists. Pediatrics 2003; 112: 1083–1087.

8   Mukohara K, Stevens DL, Schwartz M. Headache. In *Telephone Medicine: A Guide for the Practicing Physician*. Reisman AB, Stevens DL, eds. Philadelphia: American College of Physicians, 2002; pp. 199–211.

9   The Comptroller and Auditor General. *NHS Direct in England*. London: The Stationery Office, 2002.

10   O'Cathain A, Munro JF, Nicholl JP, Knowles E. How helpful is NHS Direct? Postal survey of callers. *British Medical Journal* 2000; **320**: 1035.

11   Munro J, Nicholl J, O'Cathain A, Knowles E. Impact of NHS Direct on demand for immediate care: observational study. *British Medical Journal* 2000; **321**: 150–153.

12   Brown H. NHS Direct: love it or hate it? *Geriatric Medicine* 2002; **32**: 7.

13   Atherton D. Increasing referrals are direct result of phone advice. *British Medical Association News* 2002; **7 December**: 9.

14   Richards DA, Godfrey L, Tawfik J *et al*. NHS Direct versus general practice based triage for same day appointments in primary care: cluster randomised controlled trial. *British Medical Journal* 2004; **329**: 774.

15   O'Cathain A, Webber E, Nicholl J *et al*. NHS Direct: consistency of triage outcomes. *Emergency Medical Journal* 2003; **20**: 289–292.

16   Ratcliff N. NHS Direct: help or hindrance. *Which?* 2003; **July**: 10–13.

17   Foster J, Jessopp L, Chakraborti S. Do callers to NHS Direct follow the advice to attend an accident and emergency department? *Emergency Medical Journal* 2003; **20**: 285–288.

18   Abbott J, Alberti H. NHS Direct. *British Journal of General Practice* 2001; **51**: 580–581.

19   Ullah W, Theivendra A, Sood V *et al*. Men and older people are less likely to use NHS Direct. *British Medical Journal* 2003; **326**: 710.

20   Ring F, Jones M. NHS Direct usage in a GP population of children under 5 years: is NHS Direct used by people with the greatest health need? *British Journal of General Practice* 2004; **54**: 211–213.

21   Larner AJ. Use of internet medical websites and NHS Direct by neurology outpatients before consultation. *International Journal of Clinical Practice* 2002; **56**: 219–221.

22   Larner AJ. NHS Direct: growing awareness and use. *Clinical Medicine* 2002; **2**: 275–276.

23   Larner AJ. Use of the internet and of the NHS Direct telephone helpline for medical information by a cognitive function clinic population. *International Journal of Geriatric Psychiatry* 2003; **18**: 118–122.

24   Larner AJ. NHS Direct for headache. *Journal of Neurology, Neurosurgery and Psychiatry* 2003; **74**: 1698.

25   Larner AJ. 'Self-help' for headache: NHS Direct, community pharmacists, and the internet. *Headache in Practice* 2005; in press.

▶3

Teleneurology by Email

Victor Patterson

Introduction

Email represents one of the great communication revolutions of the twentieth century. There has been enormous uptake worldwide since its first use in the early 1960s, and some people now appear to spend much of their working day simply writing email messages and replying to those from others. Within medicine, however, email has been relatively slow to catch on. There are two main ways in which email can be used medically: for doctor-to-patient interactions and for doctor-to-doctor interactions. These serve different purposes.

Doctor-to-patient email

The scope, effectiveness, acceptability and safety of doctor-to-patient email consultations have been reviewed.[1,2] The authors quote the encouragement of the Institute of Medicine[3] in the USA to use email and the Internet as a way of meeting patients' needs more responsively and at lower cost. Most published studies relate to everyday communication between patients and doctors; some doctors have used email as a method of attracting new patient referrals,[4] but others wish to stop this practice because of perceived concerns about quality, security and safety. What evidence there is suggests that these concerns are not justified.[5] Email has not yet found its niche in the routine but highly complex and varied business of patient care, but it seems likely that its use will increase gradually as suitable applications for email emerge and as both doctors and patients lose their reservations about the technique.

In neurology, Betts has documented the use of email to keep in touch with his epilepsy patients during periods when they were travelling abroad.[6] The service was used by 50 patients (however, the author does not state how many patients were offered but did not use the service). There were relatively few contacts about medical events, and most email correspondence was descriptive. There were, however, 11 contacts from foreign medical authorities asking for information about the travellers' epilepsy. Betts considered that email contact as part of 'a package of care' for travellers with epilepsy was helpful.

Presumably much unreported patient–neurologist email correspondence occurs, but it has not been subjected to scrutiny of its usefulness or its effect on neurological care.

Doctor-to-doctor email

Doctor-to-doctor email has been studied even less, and there are no systematic reviews available. Harno and colleagues compared a long-standing email referral system with conventional letter referral for patients in medical and surgical specialties referred to hospital in Finland by their general practitioners (GPs). Even though the availability of an email system stimulated demand from GPs looking for advice, the system was found to be more cost-effective than conventional referral and also had reasonable safety.[7,8] This series did not include any neurological referrals (K Harno, personal communication, 2002). Vassallo and colleagues reported a study of email-based telemedicine with multiple specialties between the Centre for the Rehabilitation of the Paralysed (CRP) in Bangladesh and specialists in the industrialized world.[9] Twenty-seven referrals were made in the first year; 70% were replied to within one day, and all were replied to within three days. The local medical staff felt that the service was beneficial to 24 of the 27 patients by (i) making a diagnosis where there was uncertainty, (ii) providing reassurance or (iii) altering management. Four patients were spared the expense of travelling abroad as a result of the telemedicine service.

There were 12 (44% of the total) neurological referrals in this series, and these have been documented in more detail;[10] eight were exceptionally complex cases and four were relatively straightforward. One of the cases reported in more detail in the appendix of the first paper had an extremely good outcome (Box 3.1) and demonstrates the potential power of teleneurology by email. Email in neurology in the developing world is described in more detail in Chapter 10.

Box 3.1 Patient CRP 009

Initial referral (patient confined to a wheelchair)
A 48-year-old, non-diabetic, normotensive, right-handed housewife presented with the following complaints: gradual weakness of both lower limbs for the past nine months, and pain in both calves. On examination of the lower limb, all tendon jerks were absent, muscle tone was reduced, and muscle power was grade III proximal and grade II in the distal group of muscles. Disease process is slowly progressive.

Initial reply
This patient seems to have a motor peripheral neuropathy. The likely cause is chronic inflammatory demyelinating peripheral neuropathy (CIDP). If you have access to nerve conduction velocities, these should be slow. Your investigations seem to have excluded myeloma and also diabetes; the other condition that needs to be excluded is lead poisoning. CIDP should respond well to steroids — prednisolone 60 mg daily is what I would use.

Further email
Following your advice, I started the patient on prednisolone. One month into the course of treatment, she is improving.

Result (after 10 emails)
The diagnosis was established, the management was changed, and the patient recovered fully and is now walking unaided.

The low-cost email telemedicine system that began at the CRP in Bangladesh is operated by a UK charity, the Swinfen Charitable Trust (SCT). Over the past few years, more and more hospitals in the developing world have referred patients by email, and at the time of writing the SCT serves about 45 hospitals in 15 countries. Neurological patients make up about 10% of referrals to the SCT; in general, they are extremely complex, and our relative success in dealing with them led us to look at the technique of email in a much simpler and more common application, that of patients referred to neurologists by GPs.[11,12] This is the subject of the rest of this chapter.

Conventional systems of referral to a neurologist

In government-provided healthcare systems such as the National Health Service (NHS) in the UK, GPs act as 'gatekeepers' for specialist services. This is both different from, and often anathema to, private-led healthcare systems, such as that of the USA, where patients can refer themselves directly to specialists. The interface between GPs and specialists in the former is therefore very important, as this type of referral can make up a considerable part of the work of neurologists. Its process is shown in Fig. 3.1.

When a GP makes a referral, he or she wants information to help manage a patient. There can be a delay in obtaining that information at any stage of the above process. If demand exceeds supply, then there may be a long waiting time for an appointment. In the UK, neurology waiting lists previously have been over two years long, but they now average about six months. This is still a very long time to wait for specialist advice about a potentially serious symptom, and it causes problems for patients, GPs, local health authorities and local politicians, who may receive letters of complaint from their constituents. It is also often dispiriting for the neurologist to see in a clinic patients who may have forgotten why they were referred in the first place. The system is in many ways unnatural, because there is effectively no dialogue between the GP and the specialist.

The basis of this communication is the posted letter, a communication method first introduced over 160 years ago. The obvious question is whether email can supplement the letter in this situation, just as it has done in many other walks of life. In other words, is email teleneurology a solution to this problem?

The advantages of email are listed in Table 3.1. The neurologist can easily enter a dialogue with the referring GP if necessary and can reply at a time and a place of his

Table 3.1. Advantages and disadvantages of email compared with communication by post

Advantages	Disadvantages
Legible	Less secure
Short and to the point	Not everyone has access
Accessible from multiple sites	
Can add attachments	
Quick to receive	
Rapid to reply	
Saves paper	

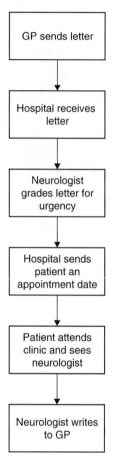

Fig. 3.1. Process of conventional letter referral.

or her choosing (Fig. 3.2). Emails tend to be briefer than letters, which are dictated and subsequently typed by secretaries, and they can take seconds rather than days to arrive.

Feasibility study of email referral

We selected nine GPs from three rural general practices in the south-west of Northern Ireland. They were located 30 minutes away by car from their local hospital and about two hours by road from the Regional Neurology Centre in Belfast (Fig. 3.3). The participating GPs not only had email on their premises but also were prepared to use it. They understood the trade-off in which patients might not be seen by a neurologist but would be guaranteed a rapid reply.

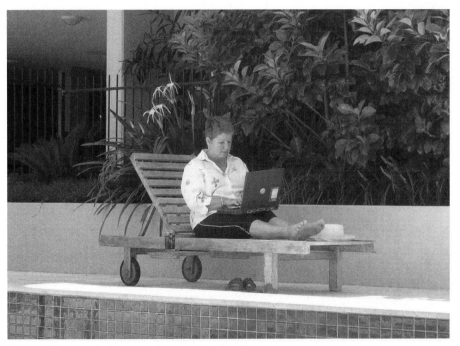

Fig. 3.2. The neurologist can reply at a convenient time.

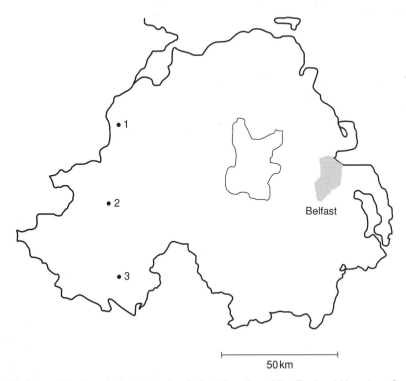

50 km

Fig. 3.3. Map of Northern Ireland, showing Belfast (location of the Regional Neurology Centre) and the location of rural practices (1, Castlederg; 2, Irvinestown; 3, Lisnaskea).

Initially, ten patients were managed by this method over three months, with no adverse events and good acceptance by both the neurologist and the GPs. The results of this pilot study showed that the system was feasible in real-life practice. We felt that a structured pro forma for the GPs to set out the details of the referral would improve the process. This was designed to be sent as an attachment to the email (Fig. 3.4).

Patient ID	Age	Sex	Occupation

Presenting symptom

History, eg duration, evolution, associated symptoms, others

Previous neurological/medical attendances to clinics

Relevant previous investigations and results

Other medical history

Drug history

Family history

Social history, eg smoking, alcohol

Examination

Pulse	BP	Fundi
Others		

Fig. 3.4. Structured pro forma sent by general practitioners as an email attachment.

Definitive study of email referral

Following the success of the feasibility study, we conducted a definitive study. This was a single-cohort design that assessed effectiveness by the reduction in the numbers of patients entering the clinic system. Satisfaction of patients and GPs was measured by questionnaires. Cost was measured by estimating the neurologist's time compared with conventional management. Safety was assessed by collecting information on adverse outcomes from the GPs' notes at least six months after completion of the telemedicine episode. We studied a consecutive cohort to glean further safety information and assess sustainability.

A summary of the email system that we used is shown in Fig. 3.5. GPs referred all consecutive patients with neurological problems in this manner. The GP sent an email using a structured pro forma to the neurologist at two different email addresses, one at the hospital and one at home. This allowed flexibility in replying and also circumvented the inevitable downtime of Internet service providers, NHS hospitals being particularly bad in this respect. The neurologist replied and (i) requested more information or (ii) arranged a clinic appointment or (iii) arranged investigations or (iv) offered advice. A copy of all email messages was sent to the neurologist's secretary, who coordinated the system. We used a protocol to ensure anonymity: each practice had a three-letter abbreviation and referrals were numbered consecutively. Thus, for example, CAS014 was the fourteenth referral from the Castlederg practice. The GP also included a unique identifying number in the subject line of the email message to enable hospital records to be tracked if a hospital appointment was necessary (see www.publications.doh.gov.uk/ipu/ahr/hrdg1802.pdf).

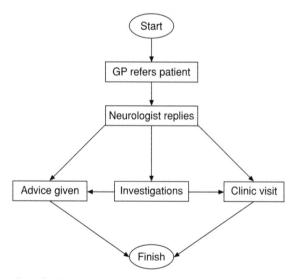

Fig. 3.5. Process of email referral.

Outcomes

Each cohort contained 76 patients, the first collected in 14 months, the second in 13. The final diagnoses from the first cohort are shown in Table 3.2. One-third of patients had structural neurological disease or epilepsy. Eighty-nine per cent of the email messages were replied to within 48 hours.

Table 3.2. Final diagnoses in the first cohort of patients (see text for details)

Final diagnosis	Total
Tension headache	18
Non-structural disease/stress	11
Uncertain	10
Epilepsy	4
Cervical radiculopathy	3
Stroke/transient ischaemic attack	3
Anxiety/panic attack	2
Carpal tunnel syndrome	2
Migraine	2
Syncope	2
Ulnar neuropathy	2
Benign positional vertigo	1
Depression	1
Horner's syndrome	1
Hypoglycaemia	1
Meralgia paraesthetica	1
Myelopathy	1
Neuralgic amyotrophy	1
Neurodegenerative disease	1
Parkinson's disease	1
Post-lumbar-puncture headache	1
Post-stroke dysaesthesiae	1
Post-viral syndrome	1
Postural hypotension	1
Raeder's syndrome	1
Restless legs	1
Tic	1
Transient global amnesia	1
Total	*76*

Effectiveness

Further information (and, therefore, a second email message) was needed in only four patients. The number of patients managed by each of the methods from the cohorts combined is shown in Fig. 3.6. The time to episode completion is shown in Fig. 3.7, with 50% of patients having their episodes completed within five days.

Satisfaction

We surveyed only the patients given advice alone. Twenty-two (65%) of 34 replied. Satisfaction was mixed, although the majority preferred the new system (see Table 3.3). GP satisfaction was uniformly high, with 100% preferring it to the conventional letter-based referral system.

Savings in the neurologist's time

The time of the neurologist to send one email was five minutes and for a subsequent clinic consultation 25 minutes.

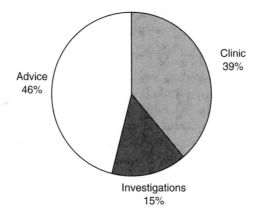

Fig. 3.6. Effectiveness of email triage (*n* = 152).

Table 3.3. Patients' responses to satisfaction questionnaire (*n* = 22)

Question	Strongly agree	Agree	Neither agree nor disagree	Disagree	Strongly disagree
1	5	3	5	6	3
2	2	9	7	2	2
3	2	10	4	1	5

Q1. I would have preferred to wait six months and see the neurologist in person.
Q2. I'm satisfied with what the neurologist said.
Q3. I would like to be dealt with in this way in the future.

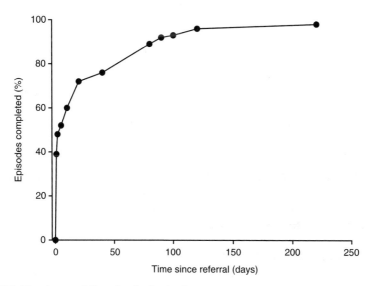

Fig. 3.7. Time to completion of patient episodes.

Time for a conventional consultation without email was taken as 30 minutes. Sixty-three patients required one email and 13 required two; the latter comprised the nine patients who needed investigations (their results were communicated to the GP by an email from the neurologist) and the four patients for whom advice alone was given but for whom the neurologist requested further information from the GP by email. The total time spent was therefore 1270 minutes (mean 16.7 minutes per patient), a reduction of 44% on the time that would have been taken had the patients been seen conventionally. Since the neurologist's time is a major factor in the cost of outpatient attendances, email triage therefore is likely to produce substantial cost savings.

Safety

A total of 152 patients were followed for a mean of 15 months. There were no deaths, 21 re-referrals and one unscheduled hospital admission. These resulted in three changes in diagnosis, all of which were minor and did not affect management.

Sustainability

It is all very well introducing new methods of practice that look good on paper, but the key test of their usefulness is whether they continue to be used after the study period has ended and the novelty has worn off. The second cohort of 76 patients was recruited in less time than the first cohort. The system has continued to be used and has been extended to 24 GPs on the basis of their expressed interest in the system rather than an active marketing campaign. The total number of referrals over the past four years is shown in Fig. 3.8.

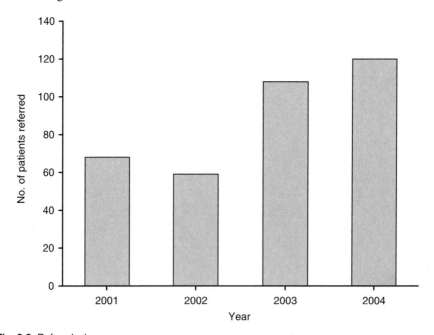

Fig. 3.8. Referrals, by year.

Customer readiness

Two theoretical objections voiced to this new system were that patients might not be happy if they were not seen physically by the specialist to whom they were referred, and similarly GPs might not be happy if their patients were not seen personally by a neurologist. In order to test these hypotheses, we identified patients who were waiting to be seen by a consulting neurologist while they were in the waiting room before their first appointment. We asked them to decide between two modes of management – one in which they would have an opinion from the neurologist quickly but would not necessarily be seen in person, and one in which the outcome would be more delayed but they would be guaranteed to be seen in person. We posed a list of similar questions to a selection of referring GPs. The responses are shown in Table 3.4. Patients were overwhelmingly positive about the new system. GPs were less enthusiastic. Nevertheless, the majority of patients and the majority of GPs were ready to use an email referral system.

Table 3.4. Preferences of patients and GPs

	n	**Email system**	**Conventional system**	**Spoilt**
Patients	100	91	8	1
GPs	85	42	40	3

Overview

Email referral certainly appears to be effective in dealing with many patients without them entering the hospital clinic system. Patients are dealt with more quickly and with less use of the neurologist's time. Acceptability by patients and GPs is good, and both patients and GPs seem ready for this novel concept.

Even though this system seems ideal, it is not for everyone. Some GPs do not have email, and some of those who do have it remain uncomfortable about using it. Many neurologists are unhappy about making a diagnosis without seeing the patient face to face. Ideally, a multi-centre trial would provide more information, but in the absence of this, there seems to be enough evidence for people interested in using email triage to do so.

The future

We have used email as a solution to two problems – reduced access to neurologists in the developing world and long waiting times to see neurologists in the industrialized world. Our problems, however, may not be everyone's, and even if they are, email may not be a feasible solution in other healthcare environments. Email is bound to have an increasing effect on neurological practice both between doctors and patients and between doctors and other doctors. This change is likely to occur gradually and inexorably in the same way that the use of multimedia projection has taken over from overhead slide projectors at academic meetings in the past 10 years. Email has the potential to make medical and neurological care less visit-based and more of a system based on continuous healing relationships and therefore may help realize one of the Institute of Medicine's simple rules for twenty-first-century healthcare.[3]

Further information

Living Internet. Electronic mail. http://livinginternet.com/e/e.htm. Accessed 25 January 2005.

References

1 Car J, Sheikh A. Email consultations in health care: 1 – scope and effectiveness. *British Medical Journal* 2004; **329**: 435–438.

2 Car J, Sheikh A. Email consultations in health care: 2 – acceptability and safe application. *British Medical Journal* 2004; **329**: 439–442.

3 Committee on Quality of Health Care in America IoM. *Crossing the Quality Chasm: A New Health System for the 21st Century.* Washington, DC: National Academies Press, 2001.

4 Borowitz SM, Wyatt JC. The origin, content, and workload of e-mail consultations. *Journal of the American Medical Association* 1998; **280**: 1321–1324.

5 Sittig DF. Results of a content analysis of electronic messages (email) sent between patients and their physicians. *BMC Medical Informatics and Decision Making* 2003; **3**: 11.

6 Betts T. Pre-departure counselling and an email contact service for patients with epilepsy faring abroad for long periods of time. *Seizure* 2004; **13**: 139–141.

7 Harno KS. Telemedicine in managing demand for secondary-care services. *Journal of Telemedicine and Telecare* 1999; **5**: 189–192.

8 Harno K, Paavola T, Carlson C, Viikinkoski P. Patient referral by telemedicine: effectiveness and cost analysis of an Intranet system. *Journal of Telemedicine and Telecare* 2000; **6**: 320–329.

9 Vassallo DJ, Hoque F, Roberts MF *et al.* An evaluation of the first year's experience with a low-cost telemedicine link in Bangladesh. *Journal of Telemedicine and Telecare* 2001; **7**: 125–138.

10 Patterson V, Hoque F, Vassallo D *et al.* Store-and-forward teleneurology in developing countries. *Journal of Telemedicine and Telecare* 2001; **7** (suppl. 1): 52–53.

11 Patterson V, Humphreys J, Chua R. Email triage of new neurological outpatient referrals from general practice. *Journal of Neurology, Neurosurgery and Psychiatry* 2004; **75**: 617–620.

12 Patterson V, Humphreys J, Chua R. Teleneurology by email. *Journal of Telemedicine and Telecare* 2003; **9** (suppl. 2): 42–43.

▶4

Teleneurology by Videoconferencing

John Craig

Introduction

There are three essential components of a successful neurological consultation: (i) a detailed and structured history from the patient and other relevant individuals; (ii) a thorough neurological and general examination; and (iii) review of any relevant investigations. Any telemedicine system that deals successfully with all of these will need to transfer large quantities of different types of information (eg audio, still images, video images) between sites. Real-time telemedicine using videoconferencing equipment offers a potential means of doing this.

Videoconferencing is the technique whereby individuals in different locations are able to communicate with each other in real time, making use of both video images and audio. In other words, the various parties are able to both see and hear each other as events take place. The result is that interaction in real time is possible (Fig. 4.1), so a true dialogue can take place.

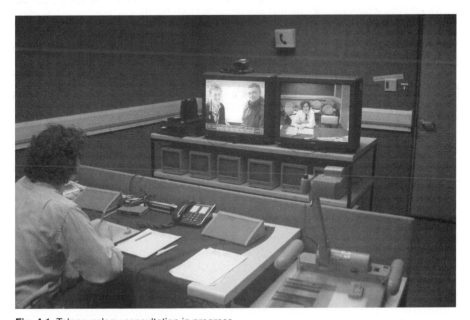

Fig. 4.1. Teleneurology consultation in progress.

Technical requirements

The technology required to undertake videoconferencing for telemedicine applications can be divided into three categories:

▶ equipment to capture the clinical information at each site

▶ communications equipment to transmit this information between the sites

▶ equipment to display the information at each site.

Commercially available videoconferencing units provide the most straightforward method of transmitting video pictures and sound for the majority of applications. A wide range of largely compatible videoconferencing equipment and accessories is now available. One benefit of using commercial suppliers is the level of support that they can provide, which includes helping to set up the system and helping to sort out technical problems as they occur. This is discussed in more detail in Chapter 12.

Initially, videoconferencing equipment was large, expensive to buy and run, and complicated to operate. Miniaturization has made it possible to develop cheaper and smaller units that can be moved between different rooms in a building. These units generally deliver high-quality video pictures on large display monitors and with high-quality sound. Further miniaturization has resulted in desktop units, which incorporate screen, camera and processor into a single piece of equipment. Most recently, the 'set-top box' has been developed in which all of the components, except the display screen, are integrated into a single unit that sits on top of a standard television (see Figs 12.1 and 12.2 in Chapter 12).

Most videoconferencing equipment is connected by digital telecommunication lines, eg integrated services digital network (ISDN) lines. Wireless units have also been developed, which use radio transmission to a nearby base station; this makes the equipment mobile. An example from paediatric practice is shown in Fig. 4.2.

Software is available to enable personal computers (PCs) to be used for videoconferencing; this should reduce the cost and expand the number of ways in which videoconferencing can be done.[1] The merits of these different systems for performing videoconferencing are summarized in Table 4.1. There should be available a system that meets most clinical needs.

Table 4.1. Types of videoconferencing system

System type	Quality of video/audio	Cost	Usage
Studio	High	High	Large group
Portable/roll-about	High	High	Small group
Set-top	High	Medium	Small group
Desktop	Medium	Medium/low	Personal
Wireless	Medium	High	Small group, mobile
Low-bandwidth (PSTN)	Low	Low	Personal

PSTN, public switched telephone network.

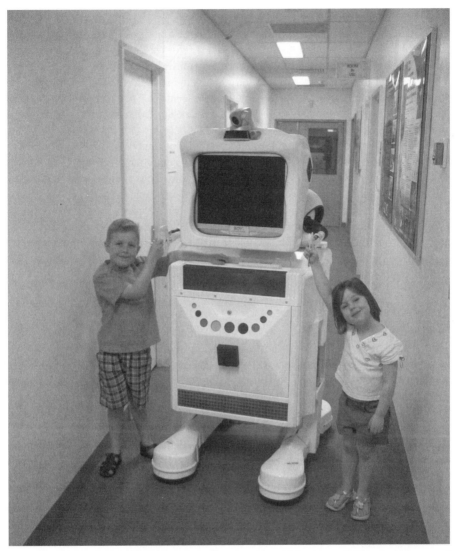

Fig. 4.2. Mobile videoconferencing system for use on a children's ward. Photograph courtesy of R Wootton.

Why consider videoconferencing?

There are two main situations when telemedicine should be used:

▶ when there is no alternative to telemedicine

▶ when telemedicine is better than existing conventional services.

When there is no alternative

In the UK, for example, the number of neurologists is grossly insufficient to deal with all patients presenting to secondary care with neurological problems. As a result, many patients are managed by doctors with little or no postgraduate training in neurology. Furthermore, traditionally, most neurologists have been based in university teaching hospitals in large population centres. Therefore if more patients are to be seen by neurologists, then it will be necessary either to greatly increase the number of neurologists and to change their usual base, or to bring all patients to the neurological centres, which will often mean the patients having to travel large distances. While there are arguments in favour of centralizing services, this idea is not supported greatly by the population as a whole. Thus, unless neurologists are willing to spend their time travelling between various hospitals (with the consequent time and cost implications), or healthcare providers are prepared to move the patients – and the patients are prepared to move – to the neurological centre, or there is a massive investment in the number of neurologists, then the only alternative for providing expert neurological care to more patients with neurological conditions is to use telemedicine.

When telemedicine is better

Telemedicine is preferable to the status quo when it provides a means by which specialists can be linked to distant patients to provide the best care available. Of course, implicit in this is the assumption that neurologists manage neurological patients more effectively than do non-neurologists. Perhaps surprisingly, information is rather limited on this point. In one study, patients presenting with neurological symptoms to outpatient departments had fewer tests, fewer referrals to other specialists and fewer review appointments when they were seen by neurologists rather than by general physicians.[2] Another observational study showed that inefficiencies might also be present in the inpatient setting.[3] The authors reported that of 75 patients who had presented with neurological symptoms to the emergency department of a large teaching hospital, 27 were admitted for further treatment. They speculated that admission might have been avoided for 10 (37%) of these patients if they had been seen by a neurologist. In a further study in the same hospital, the introduction of a liaison neurology service resulted in more diagnoses being made and shorter lengths of hospital stay for patients who had been admitted because of neurological symptoms or conditions, compared with a cohort studied a few months earlier who did not have access to this service.[4]

Thus, improved access to neurologists is likely to improve the care of patients with neurological conditions. Telemedicine offers the potential to facilitate this when distance is an issue.

It is important to remember that not all neurological episodes require a full consultation, eg giving simple advice to a colleague or a patient on one aspect of patient management, or considering the results of investigations. Hence, videoconferencing will not be necessary in all cases. Chapters 2 and 3 discuss these situations.

Performing a neurological examination using videoconferencing

What evidence is there to suggest that the neurological examination in its entirety can be interpreted by a distant specialist using videoconferencing techniques? Early reports looked at specific components of the neurological examination. Hubble and colleagues[5] showed that the motor assessment could be performed at a distance by teleconferencing in nine patients with Parkinson's disease; Chaves-Carballo[6] reported that videoconferencing could be used to diagnose childhood migraine; and Viirre and colleagues[7] reported that the signs required to diagnose benign positional vertigo could be picked up using videoconferencing.

A more recent report compared the reliability of neurological examination performed by neurologists using videoconferencing equipment versus face-to-face examination performed by junior doctors.[8] Twenty-three patients were examined face-to-face by one of five junior doctors, who recorded their findings. These examinations were witnessed by neurologists using a videoconferencing link transmitting at 384 kbit/s. The gold standard was face-to-face examination performed by one of a panel of six consultant neurologists. Power, deep tendon reflexes, plantar responses, coordination, sensation, eye movements, facial strength, tongue movements, sitting balance and gait were studied. Interobserver reliabilities were evaluated using the kappa statistic. The level of agreement between face-to-face and telemedicine examinations and the gold standard are shown in Fig. 4.3. Overall examination by

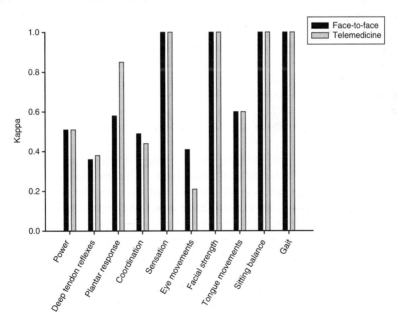

Fig. 4.3. Agreement (kappa statistic) between face-to face examination by junior doctors (black bars) and examination by telemedicine by neurology registrars (grey bars) compared with the gold standard of face-to-face examination by a panel of neurology consultants.

telemedicine compared well with face-to-face examination, being more sensitive in detecting abnormalities for all of the components of the examination studied, and more specific for all but the plantar response. Furthermore, good interobserver agreement between telemedicine observers was found. The authors emphasized that not all of the neurological examination was studied; however, others have shown that components of the examination not studied by this group can be performed, eg examination of the optic fundi has been done in screening for diabetic retinopathy,[9] and neurological examination by videoconferencing has been validated in the context of stroke assessment (see Chapter 6).[10,11]

Videoconferencing for neurological inpatients

In the development of a new telemedicine application, various steps are necessary, including:

▶ feasibility

▶ user satisfaction

▶ effectiveness.

Feasibility

In a small study from Omagh in Northern Ireland, it was shown that 25 patients who had presented with neurological symptoms could be assessed completely by distant neurologists using medium-cost videoconferencing units connected by three ISDN lines transmitting at 384 kbit/s.[12] As part of this study, all of the doctors at the remote site had been instructed on how to perform a standard examination. Overall, the median length of videoconsultation was 34 minutes, which is well within the accepted range for the normal length of a neurological consultation. The technique was learned quickly by the junior staff at the distant hospital, and extra parts of the neurological and other examination could be performed easily under the direction of the neurologist.

The feasibility of assessing patients with neurological conditions by videoconference has been reported by others. In a recent survey of US telemedicine programmes, neurology activity was fifth in terms of frequency of use by those programmes that reported their activities, coming after mental health, paediatrics, cardiology and dermatology.[13] However, because few of these programmes have published their experiences, it is unclear which types of problem are being assessed, who is assessing these patients, and how useful or otherwise the technique has been. In other neurological settings, eg stroke, the feasibility of using videoconferencing as a means of improving patient care has also been reported (see Chapter 6).

User satisfaction

Despite a substantial body of published evidence about satisfaction with telemedicine in general, information on what patients and their relatives think of being seen by a distant neurologist by videoconferencing has been studied on only a small scale. Our group from Northern Ireland reported on the satisfaction of all users (patients, neurologists, non-specialists at the rural hospital).[14] Patients reported almost universal confidence in this new method of being assessed. A small number (4/25) of patients stated that they would rather have been seen face-to-face by the neurologist, but nevertheless they felt that they had been dealt with adequately. Of note, medical staff at both sites felt confident in managing patients by this means and almost always felt that a telephone consultation would not have achieved a similarly good outcome. No major organizational difficulties were reported, and most users were satisfied with the technical aspects of the process. Overall, the findings were in keeping with high levels of reported satisfaction with other videoconferencing applications.[15] Using a similar method, Rosenthal and Schwamm report high satisfaction levels in their telestroke service (see Chapter 6.)

Effectiveness

Determining the effectiveness of any medical intervention is always a complex business. This is particularly so when one is trying to study the effect of a change in how services are delivered as part of an already established and complex healthcare system. This makes it difficult to measure the impact of teleneurology, delivered by neurologists to distant patients, using videoconferencing. As a means of overcoming this difficulty, usually different components of the application are studied. These include establishing its safety, its practicality (see above) and its utility, ie is it worthwhile? The latter may reflect clinical or financial concerns, or both.

Few studies have measured the clinical effectiveness of videoconferencing as a means of managing distant neurological patients. The outcome for some individual patients has been improved by access to distant specialists using a videolink. A woman with long-standing multiple sclerosis who had presented with unexplained coma to her local hospital had a videoconsultation with a distant neurological centre.[16] The initial working diagnosis at the local hospital was of encephalopathy secondary to a urinary tract infection. After the videolink, however, the patient was transferred to the regional neurology centre, where she was diagnosed by electroencephalography as having non-convulsive status epilepticus, which was treated successfully and from which she made a full recovery. In another paper, the same group reported the case of a man who had a history of excessive alcohol intake and who had developed acute onset of unsteadiness and weakness after a fall the preceding evening.[17] The admitting team in the rural hospital had diagnosed a posterior circulation stroke, but this was changed to acute cervical cord compression after a videolink with a distant neurologist, because of the detection of clinical signs that had been missed by the admitting medical team. Subsequent magnetic resonance imaging (MRI) of the cervical cord showed cord compression due to a prolapsed disc, which was treated neurosurgically to good effect. This latter case in particular emphasizes that in the real clinical setting, a doctor with neurological training can assess patients with neurological problems more effectively than can a less experienced doctor examining the patient face-to-face. It also illustrates the potential problems with trying to make diagnoses and plan management based on information given by distant doctors to specialists using the telephone. While this may be sufficient sometimes, this case illustrates that the neurologist, if contacted by telephone about this patient, would probably have made the wrong diagnosis and planned the wrong treatment, to the detriment of the patient.

In an attempt to measure the utility of teleneurology performed by videoconferencing, Craig and colleagues[18] undertook a cohort study comparing the management of patients admitted to two small rural hospitals that did not have neurologists on site. In one hospital, all patients presenting over a 24-week period with neurological symptoms had the option of being seen by a distant neurologist using a videolink. The sites were connected using three ISDN lines transmitting at 384 kbit/s and used commercially available videoconferencing units. In the other hospital, patients were managed as usual, ie by general physicians who could access whatever services they felt were necessary. The main outcome measure was length of hospital stay at the two hospitals for patients who had presented with neurological symptoms. The use of hospital and other healthcare resources after the patients had been discharged was also compared. As an estimate of safety, the number of times that patients had their diagnosis changed was estimated. During the study period, there were 164 patients in the intervention group, of whom 111 (68%) had a videolink. There were 128 patients in the control group. Hospital stay was significantly shorter for those patients who had access to a distant neurologist using a videolink (hazard ratio 1.13, 95% confidence interval 1.00–1.28, $p = 0.045$).

There were no differences in the use of hospital- and community-based resources between the groups. This showed that earlier discharge from hospital was not possible simply because neurologists did more investigations and did not result in additional workload for community-based services. In fact, both the number of patients undergoing a computed tomography (CT) scan and the number of patients transferred to another hospital were lower in the hospital that had a videolink. Interestingly, while the numbers of patients having arranged follow-up outpatient appointments were similar between the two groups, the type of specialist who performed the follow-up appointments was significantly different between the groups. Many more of the patients admitted to the hospital that had access by videolink to a neurologist were, not surprisingly, followed up by a neurologist. Such a shift is to be encouraged, since patients with chronic neurological conditions and who were not under the care of a neurologist were identified in the study. While it might be assumed that these patients would all be referred to a neurologist, the small number in the control group where this was actually done (2%) demonstrates that this would not be usual practice in the area in which the study was conducted. No patients who had a videolink had their diagnosis changed subsequently, in contrast to 2% of those admitted to the hospital that did not have a videolink. While the length of follow-up was short (three months), this gave some reassurance that patients could be managed safely at a distance using telemedicine. A subsequent study published in abstract form showed reasonable safety in a cohort of 221 patients followed for at least six months.[19]

The cohort comparison study, while conducted in a 'real-life' setting, illustrates the difficulties of performing clinical trials in telemedicine. In medical research, the randomized controlled trial is the gold standard by which other methodologies are compared. However, it is difficult to perform such trials in telemedicine, since the intervention itself is likely to change practice. In order to overcome this, it would be necessary to include multiple hospitals: from one half, patients would be chosen at random to have the intervention; from the other half, a random number would be chosen to be studied, having been managed as usual. When one is dealing with such a heterogeneous group of individuals as patients admitted to hospital with neurological symptoms, trying to represent fairly the multitude of potential diagnoses matched for baseline characteristics would be almost impossible. Hence, while the results from cohort studies should be scrutinized carefully, it does not seem likely that methodologically superior studies can be performed in future.

Real-time teleneurology has been used at an international level to overcome staff shortages, as reported from Australia[20]. This paper described how a neurologist in Brisbane (at 12.20 local time) was able to have a videoconference with a patient who had presented with acute headache to a small hospital in Enniskillen, Northern Ireland (at 03.20 local time). While this was undertaken only to assess feasibility, the authors postulated that such outsourcing of neurological expertise could be cost-efficient in providing out-of-hours cover.

Finally, real-time videoconferencing is effective in enabling timely administration of intravenous tissue plasminogen activator to patients with acute cerebral infarction (see Chapter 6).

Outpatient teleneurology and videoconferencing

Much of the work involving videoconferencing in neurology has concerned inpatients. However, Chua and colleagues[21] reported the results of a randomized controlled trial that studied whether new patients referred to neurological outpatient departments could be managed as efficiently, and with similar levels of acceptance, by telemedicine as by conventional face-to-face consultations. Two identical medium-cost videoconferencing units were linked using ISDN lines transmitting at 384 kbit/s. One-hundred and sixty-eight patients were studied; 86 were randomized to be seen by a distant neurologist using telemedicine, and 82 were seen face-to-face by a neurologist. The baseline characteristics and final diagnoses were similar in the two groups. Overall, levels of patient satisfaction were similar. Similar numbers in each group were offered review appointments and were prescribed medications, but the number of investigations was increased greatly in those who were seen by telemedicine. A cost analysis, including all costs incurred (staff, travel, cost of communications) showed that the average cost of a telemedicine consultation was 46% greater than conventional care [(£72 (US$135) versus £49 (US$92)].[22] However, in a subsequent study, the same authors found that the number of investigations in the telemedicine group approximated more closely to actual practice, with the investigation numbers for the face-to-face group being much lower than in usual clinical practice.[23] Videoconferencing therefore may be an economically viable means of managing distant new patients attending a neurological outpatient department.

Videoconferencing has also been used to augment nurse-led, neurologist-supported services.[24] In this report, patients with epilepsy were seen at the outpatient departments of two small rural hospitals, each of which was situated about 120 km from the neurology centre. Patients were seen by the nurse, with contact being made with the neurologist by telephone initially if there were unresolved issues regarding the consultation. Only if there were further issues was a videolink consultation with the neurologist arranged. Over the course of the study, the number of patients seen by the nurse rose from 214 in 2001 to 365 in 2003, while the number of patients needing to be seen by videolink fell from 23% to 13%. Overall, the patients were satisfied with the system, which was estimated to save the neurologist about 80% of the time that would have been required to service the conventional system. Videoconferencing has also been applied to rehabilitation in an outpatient setting (see Chapter 7).

Conclusion

The evidence in the literature shows that neurological consultation by videoconferencing can be applied to the large numbers of neurological patients, in both outpatient and inpatient settings, who because of either insufficient numbers of neurologists or geographical constraints would never have access to specialist care. The challenge now is how to plan for its widespread implementation. As Wootton[25] has described, this will also involve assessing the major structural changes required within organizations to incorporate this method of delivering healthcare, and developing 'a process for training, formulation of practice guidelines, quality control and continuing audit'. Changing the thinking of neurologists and distant physicians is, however, likely to remain one of the biggest challenges. Convincing them that the introduction of such techniques will improve patient care and, probably more importantly, be to their benefit will also be crucial. Fortunately, convincing other users, most importantly the recipients of the process, is likely to be less of a challenge.

Further information

Webster J. Desktop videoconferencing: experiences of complete users, wary users, and non-users. *MIS Quarterly* 1998; **22**: 257–286.

Wootton R, Craig J, eds. *Introduction to Telemedicine*. London: Royal Society of Medicine Press, 1999.

References

1   Falconer J. Telemedicine systems and telecommunications. In Wootton R, Craig J, eds. *Introduction to Telemedicine*. London: Royal Society of Medicine Press, 1999; pp. 17–36.

2   Patterson VH, Esmonde TF. Comparison of the handling of neurological outpatient referrals by general physicians and a neurologist. *Journal of Neurology, Neurosurgery and Psychiatry* 1993; **56**: 830.

3   Craig J, Patterson V, Rocke L, Jamison J. Accident and emergency neurology: time for a reappraisal? *Health Trends* 1997; **3**: 89–91.
4   Forbes R, Craig J, Callender M, Patterson V. Liaison neurology for acute neurological admissions. *Clinical Medicine* 2004; **4**: 290.
5   Hubble JP, Pawha R, Michalek DK *et al*. Interactive video conferencing: a means of providing interim care to Parkinson's disease patients. *Movement Disorders* 1993; **8**: 380–382.
6   Chaves-Carballo E. Diagnosis of childhood migraine by compressed interactive video. *Kansas Medicine* 1992; **93**: 353.
7   Viirre E, Warner D, Balch D, Nelson JR. Remote medical consultation for vestibular disorders: technological solutions and a case report. *Telemedicine Journal* 1997; **3**: 53–58.
8   Craig JJ, McConville JP, Patterson VH, Wootton R. Neurological examination is possible using telemedicine. *Journal of Telemedicine and Telecare* 1999; **5**: 177–181.
9   Owens DR. Telemedicine in screening and monitoring of diabetic eye disease. *Journal of Telemedicine and Telecare* 1997; **3** (suppl. 1): 89–90.
10   Wang S, Lee SB, Pardue C *et al*. Remote evaluation of acute ischemic stroke: reliability of National Institutes of Health Stroke Scale via telestroke. *Stroke* 2003; **34**: e188–191.
11   Shafqat S, Kvedar JC, Guanci MM *et al*. Role for telemedicine in acute stroke: feasibility and reliability of remote administration of the NIH stroke scale. *Stroke* 1999; **30**: 2141–2145.
12   Craig J, Patterson V, Russell C, Wootton R. Interactive videoconsultation is a feasible method for neurological in-patient assessment. *European Journal of Neurology* 2000; **7**: 699–702.
13   Grigsby B. *2004 TRC Report on US Telemedicine Activity*. Kingston, NJ: Civic Research Institute, 2004.
14   Craig J, Russell C, Patterson V, Wootton R. User satisfaction with realtime teleneurology. *Journal of Telemedicine and Telecare* 1999; **5**: 237–241.
15   Mair F, Whitten P. Systematic review of studies of patient satisfaction with telemedicine. *British Medical Journal* 2000; **320**: 1517–1520.
16   Patterson V, Craig J, Pang KA, Wootton R. Successful management of unexplained coma by telemedicine. *Journal of Telemedicine and Telecare* 1999; **5**: 134–136.
17   Patterson VH, Craig JJ, Wootton R. Effective diagnosis of spinal cord compression using telemedicine. *British Journal of Neurosurgery* 2000; **14**: 552–554.
18   Craig J, Chua R, Russell C *et al*. A cohort study of early neurological consultation by telemedicine on the care of neurological inpatients. *Journal of Neurology, Neurosurgery and Psychiatry* 2004; **75**: 1031–1035.
19   Patterson V, Chua R, Evans H, Russell C. Safety of real time telemedicine for acute neurology. *Journal of Neurology, Neurosurgery and Psychiatry* 2002; **73**: 234.
20   Patterson V, Conneally P. Intercontinental telemedicine for acute neurology. *Journal of Telemedicine and Telecare* 2005; **11**: in press.
21   Chua R, Craig J, Wootton R, Patterson. Randomised controlled trial of telemedicine for new neurological outpatient referrals. *Journal of Neurology, Neurosurgery and Psychiatry* 2001; **71**: 63–66.
22   Chua R, Craig, J, Wootton R, Patterson V. Cost implications of outpatient teleneurology. *Journal of Telemedicine and Telecare* 2001; **7** (suppl. 1): 62–64.
23   Chua R, Craig J, Esmonde T *et al*. Telemedicine for new neurological outpatients: putting a randomized controlled trial in the context of everyday practice. *Journal of Telemedicine and Telecare* 2002; **8**: 270–273.
24   Bingham E, Patterson V. A nurse led epilepsy clinic supported by telemedicine is feasible, acceptable, efficient and sustainable. *Epilepsia* 2004; **45** (suppl. 7): 52.
25   Wootton R. Telemedicine in the National Health Service. *Journal of the Royal Society of Medicine* 1998; **91**: 614–621.

Section 2: Applications

▶5

Telemedicine and Epilepsy

Jeanette C Hartshorn and Karen A Rasmusson

Introduction

Telemedicine can be used successfully to treat many neurological diseases[1-3]. Despite little work having been carried out in the area of epilepsy, this disorder appears to be highly suitable for management by telemedicine. Epilepsy is common. A 50-year study based on the Rochester (Minnesota) Epidemiology Project estimated that approximately 10% of the US population has suffered from some type of convulsive disorder.[4] Most studies show that the prevalence of epilepsy is about one in 200 people.

Epilepsy causes transportation problems because the affected individual may not be able to drive if they continue to have seizures. This results in sporadic care, which in turn can lead to an increase in the severity of the patient's seizures and a decrease in medication compliance. The use of telemedicine should lessen this problem by reducing the need for patients to travel. In addition, when the clinic is closer to home, a patient is more likely to be accompanied by family members. This is important, because family members can provide valuable information about the patient's behaviour and symptoms during seizures[5,6]. Without such corroboration, the healthcare provider may not receive a full picture of the patient's problems.

Previous studies

A MEDLINE search in February 2005 for studies about telemedicine and epilepsy found 12 publications on the subject; when the use of the telephone and email was excluded, there were only seven publications. Many physicians and patients use email as a common form of communication,[5,7,8] so it is perhaps surprising that there is only a single report of its use in epilepsy.

There is a single report of a nurse-led epilepsy clinic supported by telemedicine[9] and a single report of the use of videoconferencing to deliver counselling to adolescents with epilepsy and psychosocial adjustment problems.[10] We have used telemedicine for five years in the management of patients with epilepsy. This service developed as a partnership between the University of Texas Medical Branch (UTMB) at Galveston, the Texas Department of Health (TDH) and the Epilepsy Foundation of Southeast Texas (EFSET).

University of Texas Medical Branch

The UTMB is a large academic medical centre that treats patients from Texas, from America in general and from around the world. In 2004, there were more than 35 000 inpatient admissions and more than 850 000 outpatient visits. The UTMB began using telemedicine to provide healthcare to inmates of the Texas correctional care system in 1994. The UTMB Telehealth Center promotes the use of technology for patient- and family-focused care. It also provides other institutions with assistance in developing and implementing telemedicine and distance education programmes. The UTMB has a particular interest in caring for special populations, including women and children, indigent people, elderly people and incarcerated people.[11,12] The telemedicine programme conducts an average of 4000 telemedicine visits per month. It was the most active telemedicine network of those surveyed recently by the Telemedicine Information Exchange.[13]

Epilepsy Foundation of Southeast Texas

The EFSET is a non-profit-making organization founded in 1983 to improve the lives of the almost 100 000 adults and children with epilepsy in south-east Texas. In 2000, EFSET joined with the TDH to start a programme for people with epilepsy who are uninsured and ineligible for Medicaid or Medicare (US government insurance programmes). These patients are often described as the 'working poor', since they frequently have some income, making them ineligible for most government insurance schemes even though they are unable to afford healthcare.

The TDH programme was intended to bring care to these individuals and to maximize their opportunities to continue to work. The telemedicine clinics provide medical, psychosocial, educational and employment services. There is evidence that this approach is effective. In 2003, over 90% of EFSET patients reported a reduction in seizure frequency and improved quality of life.[14]

Clinic location

There are an estimated 47 000 people with epilepsy in the south-east Texas region. Twenty-six of the 36 counties in this region are designated as completely or partially medically underserved areas (MUAs), so there are few resources for people with epilepsy.

The UTMB provides epilepsy clinics by telemedicine from a central site in Galveston to two peripheral clinics in Beaumont and Houston (Fig. 5.1). Weekly telemedicine epilepsy clinics are held in Beaumont, with an average of 12–14 patients per clinic. Monthly clinics are held in Houston, with an average of 8–10 patients per clinic.

Without the telemedicine epilepsy clinic in Beaumont, patients would have to travel 160 km in each direction to see their doctor at the UTMB, with the accompanying

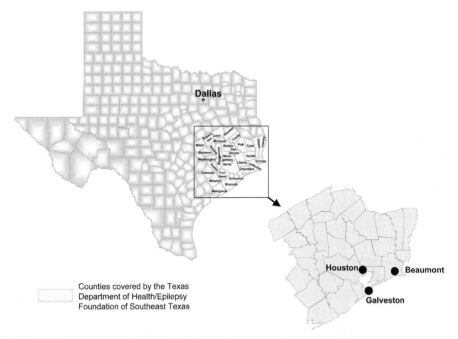

Counties covered by the Texas
Department of Health/Epilepsy
Foundation of Southeast Texas

Fig. 5.1. Texas Department of Health/Epilepsy Foundation of Southeast Texas coverage.

problems of transportation costs and time off work. Patients also receive discounted diagnostic testing and medication assistance through the clinics.[15]

Staff

The Beaumont telemedicine epilepsy clinic began seeing patients in 2000. Staffing for the clinics includes a neurologist, an advanced practice nurse (APN) who specializes in the treatment of epilepsy, a nurse presenter and a programme coordinator. The neurologist and the APN in Galveston see patients and are assisted by a nurse presenter. The nurse presenter functions as an amanuensis for the healthcare provider. In preparation for this, the nurse will have trained with the neurologist. The nurse assists the provider with the physical examination, using a document camera or electronic stethoscope if necessary.

An important part of the success of these clinics is the use of a case-management model of care, which ensures continuity of care delivery. The programme coordinators schedule visits and diagnostic testing, track medication, collect statistics for the TDH reports and communicate with patients. They help patients to take full advantage of the patient-assistance programmes offered by the major pharmaceuticals companies. In one year, they were able to obtain US$135 000 (£72 000) worth of medication. Patients have expressed favourable opinions about the telemedicine clinics (Box 5.1).

Box 5.1 Patients' opinions about telemedicine clinics

'Always they are just as good as gold. They take care of me. They are all wonderful folks.'

'Without the telemedicine clinic, I would not be here today. My husband's plant [place of work] was closed after 30 years of insurance. I had nowhere to go and no money. The clinic people helped me get prescriptions I had been without for four months.'

'My husband and I are on a very small limited income. If it were not for the telemedicine clinic, I couldn't afford to take the anticonvulsants I need each day. They are very expensive.'

Procedure

Patients are provided with a detailed overview of telemedicine and the clinic's services when they arrive at the clinic. Each patient signs a consent form for treatment as well as a special consent form for telemedicine services. All sessions are held in an examination room with acoustic measures to maintain confidentiality. The nurse presenter explains the telemedicine procedure (Fig. 5.2).

In our and others' experience,[16–18] a comprehensive neurological examination is normally possible using telemedicine. Cranial nerve examinations, mental status, extraocular movements, reflexes and cerebellar testing can all be accomplished using

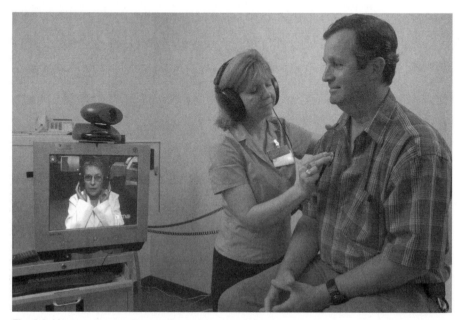

Fig. 5.2. Nurse presenter with a patient at the remote clinic.

telemedicine. Sensory testing can also be done using telemedicine, although occasionally it is necessary to bring the patient to the UTMB for more detailed testing. During the consultation, the nurse presenter is available to answer the patient's questions and deal with the patient's concerns. If the patient wishes to have a private conversation with the provider, then the nurse leaves the room and returns when requested by the patient.

Telemedicine system

A healthcare provider at the central site (Fig. 5.3) communicates with a presenter and the patient at a remote site via the telemedicine link. The central site (UTMB) and the remote site (Beaumont) have similar videoconferencing equipment. In Beaumont, it is housed in a roll-about cabinet with a 43-cm flat-screen monitor (Fig. 5.4). The cabinet can hold a range of medical instrumentation. The videoconferencing units are connected by integrated services digital network (ISDN) lines at a bandwidth of 384 kbit/s, which provides good-quality video pictures at both sites.[19]

Digital encryption is used to ensure the security of the patient information. Images, such as magnetic resonance scans, can be accessed at the central site via a separate computer (Fig. 5.5). A fax machine is used to transmit patient information, such as a prescription from the provider.

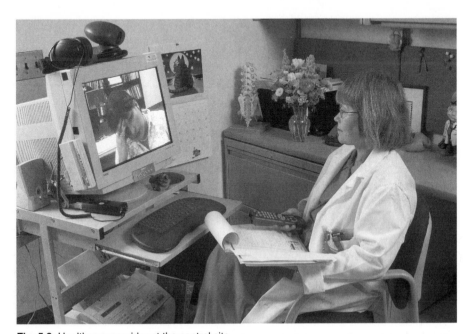

Fig. 5.3. Healthcare provider at the central site.

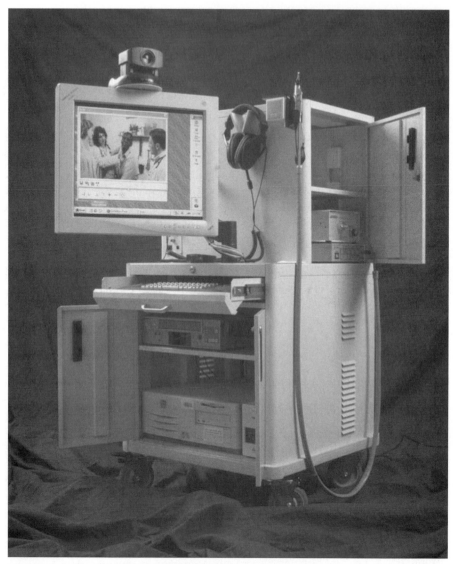

Fig. 5.4. Roll-about telemedicine cabinet at the remote clinic.

Outcomes

We have conducted a comparison of telemedicine care with traditional care. We surveyed patients at a telemedicine clinic and at a traditional ambulatory clinic. Data on 155 patients from the two clinics (Beaumont, telemedicine, $n = 83$; Galveston, traditional, $n = 72$) were collected during a three-month period in 2004.[20] The principal outcome measures were the numbers of seizures, hospitalizations and emergency-

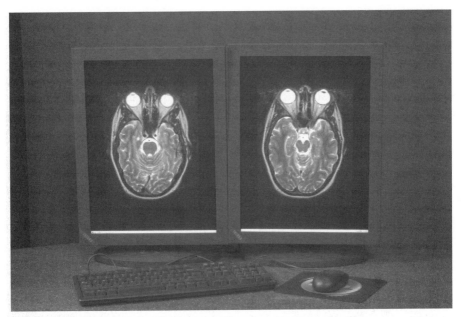

Fig. 5.5. Image-viewing station showing magnetic resonance image of brain.

room visits. We also assessed medication compliance using both self-report and medication levels. Information on laboratory work and diagnostic testing, information and referrals, patient encounters and medication was also gathered.

The age and marital status data of the subjects were similar in both clinics. The average age of the women and men was 56 and 45 years, respectively. Single or divorced subjects accounted for 58% of those studied; 38% were married or widowed. Ethnicity was slightly different in the two groups due to the population differences between the two catchment areas.

There was no significant difference in any of the outcome measures between the two groups (Table 5.1). Thus, there was no evidence to suggest that a telemedicine clinic is in any way inferior to a traditional face-to-face clinic for patients with epilepsy. An example showing the power of the telemedicine service is given on page 50.

Table 5.1. Outcome measures (mean values) in the two groups

	Beaumont (telemedicine) ($n=83$)	Galveston (control) ($n=72$)	Difference p
Seizures (n)	4.8	4.6	>0.05
Emergency-room visits (n)	8	9	>0.05
Hospitalizations (n)	2	9	>0.05
Medication compliance (%)	82	88	>0.05

Case report

Mr T is a 28-year-old developmentally delayed African-American male with a history of complex partial seizures with secondary generalization since birth. He has been taking carbamazepine for many years. He lives at home with his parents and works during the week at a sheltered workshop. Before the opening of the Beaumont Telemedicine Clinic, Mr T was seen annually in Galveston. His father brought him to each visit and always reported that his son had been seizure-free with no significant problems over the past year. During the interview, the patient was noted to rock back and forth in his chair and frequently carried on conversations with himself. At times, the patient seemed agitated. In spite of these observations, his father always assured the APN that this was normal behaviour and that it caused no problems for his son at work or at home.

As Mr T lives in Beaumont, he was transferred to the telemedicine clinic once it opened. Since the clinic was much closer to his home, he was then accompanied to the clinic by his mother. She reported that Mr T was 'a handful', particularly with relation to his behaviour. His difficulties with impulse control and lack of anger management caused problems at work and home. She explained that his father was absent most of the time. In addition, the father never communicated with the workshop about his son.

Although Mr T's problems were discussed by his parents, the father had limited first-hand knowledge of the problems and, thus, never reported any difficulties. The patient's mother was under the impression that her husband was reporting these events to the APN. Due to her own ill health, Mr T's mother was unable to drive her son to Galveston; with the clinic closer to their home, she was able to accompany her son and participate actively in each visit.

Based on the insights of the patient's mother, Mr T was started on a low dosage of an antipsychotic medication, which stopped most of his disruptive behaviour without increasing his seizures. The management of his care was improved greatly through telemedicine. Although the information provided by the patient's mother could have been obtained via telephone, there was no indication from his father that additional information was available or relevant.

As this case illustrates, it is important to ensure that the primary caregivers of a person with developmental disabilities are involved in the patient's medical care. In this case, telemedicine provided an opportunity for the involvement that was not readily available with more traditional treatment models.

Limitations

Our experience is that the appropriate infrastructure must be in place for the successful practice of telemedicine. Appropriate training on all the equipment for all those involved is absolutely essential, as are skilled technical people to maintain and troubleshoot equipment operations.[21] In addition, diagnostic testing must be available near to where the patient lives, otherwise telemedicine will lose much of its advantage.

A problem for telemedicine practice in the USA is the lack of reimbursement by some insurance and government schemes. Our epilepsy project has been possible only because of grant funding and the volunteer efforts of the staff. The project shows that telemedicine is an acceptable method for delivery of comprehensive care to adults with epilepsy, especially for those patients unable to access or afford care from another venue.

The future

Having shown that telemedicine using videoconferencing is feasible in epilepsy, studies are now needed to investigate its cost-effectiveness. Such studies should take into account the benefits for patients of improved access to care and the savings from fewer emergency-room visits and hospitalizations that are associated with a better service. Another model to explore is the use of videoconferencing to link epileptologists to neurologists or primary-care providers for periodic consultation. This should allow periodic consultations and produce greater continuity of care.

Our experience suggests that telemedicine is an acceptable, effective and safe alternative to traditional face-to-face clinics for providing care to adults with epilepsy. It should be easier to organize a telemedicine service than a conventional one in rural and remote areas and for underserved populations. There are large numbers of such patients in the USA, and elsewhere, who would benefit from a telemedicine epilepsy service.

Further information

Goodwin M, Higgins S, Lanfear JH *et al*. The role of the clinical nurse specialist in epilepsy: a national survey. *Seizure* 2004; **13**: 87–94.

Heaney DC, Begley CE. Economic evaluation of epilepsy treatment: a review of the literature. *Epilepsia* 2002; **43** (suppl. 4): 10–16.

Maulden SA. Information technology, the internet, and the future of neurology. *Neurologist* 2003; **9**: 149–159.

References

1   Craig J, Chua R, Russell C *et al*. A cohort study of early neurological consultation by telemedicine on the care of neurological inpatients. *Journal of Neurology, Neurosurgery and Psychiatry* 2004; **75**: 1031–1035.
2   Chua R, Craig J, Wootton R, Patterson V. Randomised controlled trial of telemedicine for new neurological outpatient referrals. *Journal of Neurology, Neurosurgery and Psychiatry* 2001; **71**: 63–66.
3   LaMonte M, Bahouth M, Hu P *et al*. Telemedicine for acute stroke: triumphs and pitfalls. *Stroke* 2003; **34**: 725–728.
4   Hauser W, Annegers J, Rocca W. Descriptive epidemiology of epilepsy: contributions of population-based studies from Rochester, Minnesota. *Mayo Clinic Proceedings* 1996; **71**: 576–586.
5   Elger CE, Burr W. Advances in telecommunications concerning epilepsy. *Epilepsia* 2000; **41** (suppl. 5): 9–12.

6   Ottman R, Hauser WA, Susser M. Validity of family history data on seizure disorders. *Epilepsia* 1993; **34**: 469–475.

7   Prady SL, Norris D, Lester JE, Hoch DB. Expanding the guidelines for electronic communication with patients: application to a specific tool. *Journal of the American Medical Informatics Association* 2001; **8**: 344–348.

8   Betts T. Pre-departure counselling and an email contact service for patients with epilepsy faring abroad for long periods of time. *Seizure* 2004; **13**: 139–141.

9   Bingham E, Patterson V. A nurse led epilepsy clinic supported by telemedicine is feasible, acceptable, efficient and sustainable. *Epilepsia* 2004; **45** (suppl. 7): 52.

10 Glueckauf RL, Fritz SP, Ecklund-Johnson EP *et al.* Videoconferencing-based family counseling for rural teenagers with epilepsy: phase I findings. *Rehabilitation Psychology* 2002; **47**: 49–72.

11 Robinson S, Seale D, Tiernan K, Berg B. Use of telemedicine to follow special needs children. *Telemedicine Journal and e-Health* 2003; **9**: 57–61.

12 Raimer BG, Stobo JD. Health care delivery in the Texas prison system: the role of academic medicine. *Journal of the American Medical Association* 2004; **292**: 485–489.

13 Telemedicine Information Exchange. Telemedicine Programs Database. http://tie.telemed.org/programs/showprogram.asp?item=2574. Accessed 8 February 2005.

14 Epilepsy Foundation of Southeast Texas. *Report to the Texas Department of Health.* Beaumont: EFSET 2003.

15 Hartshorn JC, Rasmusson KA. A model epilepsy telemedicine clinic for underserved populations. *Telemedicine Journal and e-Health* 2002; **8**: 250.

16 Hildebrand R, Chow H, Williams C *et al.* Feasibility of neuropsychological testing of older adults via videoconference: implications for assessing the capacity for independent living. *Journal of Telemedicine and Telecare* 2004; **10**: 130–134.

17 Craig JJ, McConville JP, Patterson VH, Wootton R. Neurological examination is possible using telemedicine. *Journal of Telemedicine and Telecare* 1999; **5**: 177–181.

18 Shafqat S, Kvedar JC, Guanci MM *et al.* Role for telemedicine in acute stroke: feasibility and reliability of remote administration of the NIH stroke scale. *Stroke* 1999; **30**: 2141–2145.

19 Hartshorn JC. Primary care telemedicine: increased patient satisfaction and lower costs. *Telehealth Practice Report* 2004; **9**: 3, 15.

20 Rasmusson K, Hartshorn J. A comparison of epilepsy patients in a traditional ambulatory clinic and a telemedicine clinic. *Epilepsia* 2005, in press.

21 Yellowlees PM. Successfully developing a telemedicine system. In Wootton R, Craig J, eds. *Introduction to Telemedicine.* London: Royal Society of Medicine Press, 1999; pp. 93–103.

▶6

Telemedicine and Stroke

Eric S Rosenthal and Lee H Schwamm

Introduction

Stroke is a major cause of death and disability worldwide. Over 280 000 people in the USA die from stroke each year.[1] Most therapeutic interventions were targeted at stroke prevention until 1995, when the results of a large randomized controlled trial of intravenous (IV) tissue-type plasminogen activator (tPA) in acute ischaemic stroke documented a 4% absolute mortality benefit and a 30% increase in the likelihood of having little or no disability at follow-up.[2] Benefit, however, was restricted to patients receiving tPA within three hours of symptom onset. The protocol for tPA administration in this trial was strict but important, since adverse events were more common among patients with protocol violations. Expertise in stroke management therefore is crucial in the delivery of IV tPA, and the shortage of this expertise may explain why it has been used in less than 3% of patients with ischaemic stroke in the USA.[3] The discrepancy between the efficacy of tPA and its limited use is a significant problem that may be solved by telemedicine bringing a stroke expert to the bedside.

Current problems with access to intravenous tPA

Pre-hospital delays

Less than half of all patients with acute stroke are seen in a hospital emergency department within three hours of symptom onset.[4] Specifically, patients in remote locations and those in hospitals without stroke expertise may have limited access to thrombolysis. During a study of non-urban east Texas communities in the USA, only 1.4% of patients with ischaemic stroke received IV tPA,[5] versus 14.7% at the university hospital in the nearest major city (Houston).[6] Other studies have linked racial, ethnic, geographical and socioeconomic differences to low rates of tPA utilization,[4,6] suggesting that the populations most underserved by stroke expertise are least likely to receive tPA.

Lack of stroke expertise

Even when tPA is delivered to patients with ischaemic stroke, higher rates of adverse outcomes occur when thrombolytic therapy is delivered without consultation by physicians with specialized stroke expertise. In one study, 16% of treated patients developed symptomatic intracerebral haemorrhage (ICH) compared with 6% in the National Institute of Neurological Disorders and Stroke (NINDS) trial. Although 96% of treatment decisions involved a neurologist, deviations from NINDS guidelines were observed in 50% of treated patients.[7] Aggressive corrective measures increased the rate of tPA administration while reducing symptomatic ICH to 6% among treated patients.[8] Other studies have linked increased rates of protocol violations to increased rates of symptomatic ICH and mortality.[9,10]

Unnecessary interfacility transfers

Helicopter transport has been employed to shorten the time to presentation at large centres. Results, however, have been mixed. In one study, direct helicopter transport to a tertiary-care facility improved access to tPA but resulted in the costly transfer of patients ineligible for tPA (more than 80% of transported patients).[11] The average field-to-hospital distance for all patients was 47 km. Such transport is expensive and only transferred patients receive the benefit of a full neurological consultation. When patients are transported by helicopter *after* triage at a community hospital, the time delays become prohibitive.

Telemedicine as a solution

Real-time teleneurology, by collapsing the boundaries of time and space, can permit stroke expertise to travel instantaneously to the bedside. This enables triage, evaluation and treatment to be provided locally with a more efficient use of resources. Telemedicine-enabled support for the delivery of tPA to patients had its first success in patients with myocardial infarction: rapid delivery of tPA to patients in rural Greece was enabled after the history, physical examination and electrocardiogram (ECG) were reviewed by telephone and fax by physicians in Athens. Door-to-needle times were 20–30 minutes.[12]

The telemedicine-based evaluation of acute stroke is especially challenging. It requires a rapid neurological assessment, computed tomography (CT) image acquisition and review, and a detailed history for tPA exclusion criteria. Low-cost teleradiology systems are now available for the transmission of compressed CT images viewable on a conventional personal computer (PC) monitor, in accordance with published standards.[13,14] The decreased cost of videoconferencing equipment allows a physician with clinical and imaging stroke expertise to conduct a remote history, physical examination and radiological interpretation in real time for the purposes of diagnosing and managing patients with stroke symptoms.[15]

Establishing a telestroke service

Equipment

In our telestroke service, a videoconferencing link is established between a community hospital (emergency physician) and a tertiary-care hospital (stroke neurologist). All patients are examined on a stretcher in the community hospital's emergency department using a commercial videoconferencing system on a mobile cart (Fig. 6.1). The videoconferencing equipment (ViewStation 512, Polycom, Pleasanton, USA) is connected by three integrated services digital network (ISDN) lines (384 kbit/s) and transmits 30 frames per second. Most studies on stroke treatment have used ISDN, but some have used Internet Protocol (IP) over a virtual private network. ISDN at a bandwidth of less than 384 kbit/s has not been evaluated for acute neurological management and may not be suitable for clinical applications.

In our system, CT scans are transmitted in Digital Imaging and Communications in Medicine (DICOM) format and displayed with browser-based image software (AMICAS, Inc., Boston, USA) on a PC monitor set at a resolution of 1024×768 pixels. This permits side-by-side clinical and radiological evaluation (Fig. 6.2) by the consulting stroke neurologist.

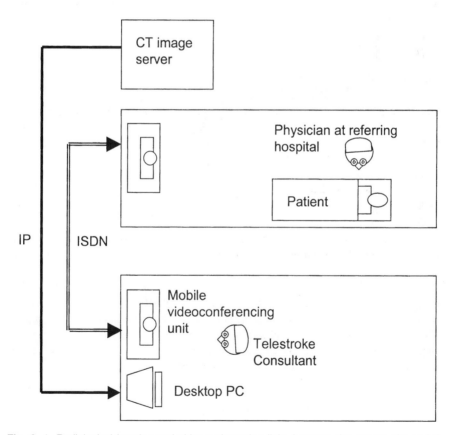

Fig. 6. 1. Radiological imaging and videoconferencing links between the remote site and the telestroke expert centre.

CT, computed tomography; IP, Internet Protocol; ISDN, integrated services digital network; PC, personal computer.

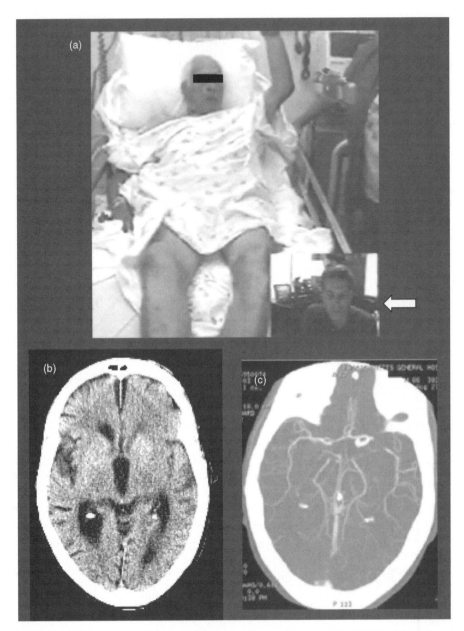

Fig. 6. 2. (a) Still frame from the telestroke examination by the neurologist at home (inset picture, white arrow) examining the patient at a remote hospital. Right face and arm weakness can be observed as the patient is asked to raise both arms and look straight ahead. (b) Non-contrast computed tomography (CT) of the brain obtained less than 30 minutes after symptom onset viewed from the remote stroke physician's home via teleradiology. Subtle signs of early ischaemia include loss of normal contour of the posterior left putamen and insular ribbon. (c) Follow-up CT angiography after transfer at four hours after symptom onset shows a persistent left middle cerebral artery occlusion.

Validating the neurological examination

Studies have compared directly the telemedicine-enabled video observations of a neurologist at 384 kbit/s with the bedside examination of a house officer and the gold standard examination of a panel of six neurologists.[16] The observations of the telemedicine-enabled neurologist were as good as the examination performed in person by the house officer and were in almost perfect agreement (kappa score 0.81–1.00) with the gold standard panel for many components of the neurological examination.

Previously, we have validated the National Institutes of Health Stroke Scale (NIHSS) assessment as a reliable method of evaluating patients with stroke symptoms,[17] using a bandwidth of 384 kbit/s. There was an excellent correlation between bedside and remote scores (inter-rater correlation coefficient 0.97, $p < 0.001$), with little increase in the time to perform the evaluation. The inter-rater agreement between telemedicine and bedside examinations was similar to that between any two bedside examinations in previous validation studies of the NIHSS.[18] The Remote Evaluation of Acute Ischemic Stroke (REACH) project validated the NIHSS in clinical practice, with an excellent correlation between a bedside and remote NIHSS score ($r = 0.96$, $p = 0.0001$).[19] In studies of stroke patients by Handschu and colleagues, weighted kappa statistics were greater than 0.85 for all aspects of NIHSS scores, except for the examination of facial paresis in patients seen within six hours of symptom onset.[20]

Radiological evaluation of transmitted images

Rapid transmission and accurate interpretation of radiological images are essential in determining eligibility for IV thrombolysis among patients with stroke symptoms. Because the accuracy of interpreting these radiological studies affects outcomes after thrombolytic therapy, the interpreter must be able to detect exclusion criteria for the administration of IV tPA. ICH on initial CT is an absolute contraindication, and some data suggest that hypodensity on acute brain CT is associated with haemorrhagic transformation after thrombolysis, especially when such a hypodensity occupies more than one-third of the middle cerebral artery territory (>1/3MCA).[2,21] The importance of early ischaemic changes (EIC), such as sulcal effacement and ventricular compression, is more controversial. CT protocol violations in thrombolytic trials have been associated with high rates of adverse events,[22] and treatment of patients in the presence of CT exclusion criteria yields excess risk with no observable benefit.[23]

Convenience sampling of emergency physicians, neurologists and radiologists suggests that neurologists have near-perfect sensitivity for detecting obvious haemorrhage but are less accurate in detecting subtle haemorrhages or hypodensities > 1/3MCA.[24] These studies, however, did not assess separately those neurologists with prior stroke training.

The low-cost teleradiology systems referred to above make it possible to distribute images without an expensive picture-archiving and communication system (PACS). In a web browser, images can be viewed on conventional PC monitors located in the hospital or the physician's home. One pilot study compared stroke neurologists' readings of CT images via teleradiology versus gold standard readings of hard copies on a viewing box. Each neurologist read half of the CT scans in a blinded fashion using teleradiology and read the other half using a viewing box. Using the official reading by a neuroradiologist as the gold standard, there was perfect agreement between groups and perfect sensitivity and specificity for the determination of tPA eligibility by the stroke neurologist.[25]

We have also validated that a telemedicine review (by a stroke neurologist) of DICOM-compressed brain CT images can identify accurately candidates for IV tPA. This is set out in more detail in Table 6.1.[26] Thus, real-time interpretation of CT scans on a PC during a telestroke consultation compares favourably with image interpretation performed on a viewing box or on a PACS workstation by neuroradiologists.

To make the process practical for community hospitals, the equipment must be inexpensive and easy to operate in an emergency department. Transmission of CT images to experienced radiologists for formal interpretation is essential for quality control and feedback. A team of experienced acute stroke specialists linked remotely by telestroke systems may thus provide on-call acute stroke consultation to multiple hospitals without each facility maintaining its own continuously available stroke consultation service with clinical and imaging expertise.

Telestroke in clinical practice

Diagnosis and management

A team at the University of Maryland reported 23 telemedicine consultations and 27 telephone consultations preceding transfer among patients with suspected acute stroke.[27] Of the 23 telemedicine consultations, two were aborted because of technical difficulties, but five of the 21 patients receiving successful telestroke consultation also received IV tPA. No patient experienced complications. Diagnoses included subarachnoid haemorrhage, ICH, seizure, hypoglycaemia and transient ischaemic attack (TIA), as well as acute ischaemic stroke (both anterior and posterior circulation).

A large series of telestroke consultations has been described in southern Germany, in which seven rural hospitals were linked to a stroke unit in Gunzburg as part of the Telemedicine in Stroke in Swabia (TESS) project.[28] Of 153 patients examined, 87 were found to have had an ischaemic stroke, but, importantly, 40 patients had a diagnosis other than stroke, confirming that telemedicine is also helpful in identifying other emergency neurological conditions. The average duration of teleconsultation was 15 minutes. Thirty-seven per cent of the 94 patients with ischaemic stroke or TIA reached the hospital within three hours, and two received thrombolysis. In the opinion of the referring physicians, relevant contributions concerning the diagnostic workup, CT assessment and therapeutic recommendations were made in over 75% of all cases.

In the REACH study among five rural hospitals in Georgia,[29] 12 out of 75 patients evaluated received tPA, all without ICH complications. Within this system, staff at the

Table 6.1. Inter-rater agreement expressed as kappa (κ) scores for 26 computed tomography (CT) scans interpreted by a stroke neurologist and a staff neuroradiologist. A neuroradiologist with stroke expertise reviewed the first 15 of these scans

CT finding	SN v. Stroke-NRAD		SN v. Staff-NRAD		Staff-NRAD v. Stroke-NRAD	
	κ	95% CI	κ	95% CI	κ	95% CI
ICH						
Conventional method	1.00	1.00, 1.00	1.00	1.00, 1.00	1.00	1.00, 1.00
Estimating equations method	1.00	1.00, 1.00	1.00	1.00, 1.00	1.00	1.00, 1.00
Acute hypodensity						
Conventional method	0.63	−0.01, 1.28	0.24	−0.28, 0.75	0.62	−0.04, 1.28
Estimating equations method	0.33*	−0.34, 0.78	0.31	−0.31, 0.75	0.33*	−0.29, 0.76
Subtle signs of acute infarct						
Conventional method	1.00	1.00, 1.00	0.54	0.15, 0.93	0.39	−0.30, 1.08
Estimating equations method	1.00	0.97, 1.00	0.36*	−0.17, 0.73	0.33	−0.27, 0.75
Any early ischaemic changes						
Conventional method	0.76	0.32, 1.20	0.29	−0.11, 0.69	0.23	−0.40, 0.86
Estimating equations method	0.82*	0.41, 0.96	0.16*	−0.30, 0.56	0.20*	−0.34, 0.64
Chronic ischaemic lesions						
Conventional method	0.88	0.59, 1.13	0.63	0.32, 0.93	0.79	0.41, 1.17
Estimating equations method	0.83	0.42, 0.96	0.62	0.19, 0.85	0.77	0.25, 0.95

CI, confidence interval; ICH, intracranial haemorrhage; SN, stroke neurologist; Staff-NRAD, staff neuroradiologist; Stroke-NRAD, neuroradiologist with stroke expertise.
*Use of an adjusted κ score changed the level of agreement.

emergency department of a rural community hospital can consult an on-call telemedicine-enabled stroke neurologist at any time of the day.

In our own telestroke experience in Massachusetts,[26] six patients were treated with IV tPA in the first 27 months. Of these, two had persistent deficits (one of whom had care withdrawn), two had moderate recovery, and two had good recovery (one of whom initially had worsening deficits). There were no violations of the NINDS protocol,[2] and no CT scans were misinterpreted. All patients had follow-up imaging, and only one patient developed symptomatic ICH within 36 hours; another developed a small late asymptomatic haemorrhage.

Thrombolytic therapy was given to 106 patients as part of the Telemedic Pilot Project for Integrative Stroke Care (TEMPiS) in Bavaria, Germany. The network consists of two comprehensive centres and 12 regional centres connected by round-the-clock telemedicine support for stroke care. In the first year following intervention, the number of patients treated with tPA increased to 86 (2% of all those admitted with stroke), compared with 10 patients treated in the year preceding intervention. The rate of symptomatic haemorrhage was 8.5%, similar to that in the NINDS trial.[30]

Efficiency of tPA administration

In the first 27 months of our telestroke experience,[26] 26 consultations were requested. Twelve of these began within three hours of symptom onset. Eight of these 12 patients had acute ischaemic stroke, of which two were not treated due to mild deficits. Three were diagnosed with TIA or migraine, and one was diagnosed with a subdural haematoma not detected at the local facility. For the 12 acute cases for which rapid diagnosis and management were essential, we determined the mean times from symptom onset to start of telestroke consultation and from consultation start to drug delivery or to determination of tPA ineligibility (Table 6.2). Similar times were achieved in the REACH system and TEMPiS.

Table 6.2. Mean time between stages of tissue-type plasminogen activator (tPA) administration in six published studies contrasting telestroke interventions (T) with conventional mechanisms of care (C). Telestroke patients were treated at a community or rural hospital by a remotely located stroke expert using videoconferencing. Patients presenting through conventional mechanisms were treated by on-site stroke physicians. Interval mean times have been interpolated if not reported specifically

Stroke centre	Patient population	Sample	Mean time (min)			
			Symptom-to-door	Door-to-consultation	Consultation-to-needle	Symptom-to-needle
Massachusetts (T)	Rural	Received tPA ($n = 6$)	36	70	36	142
REACH (T)	Rural	Received tPA ($n = 12$)	71	45	18	134
TEMPiS (T)	Rural	Received tPA ($n = 106$)	65	15	61	141
Ontario* (C)	Rural	Received tPA ($n = 23$)	34	89	49	172
Houston (C)	Urban	Received tPA ($n = 269$)	67	70		137

*The door-to-consultation time in the Ontario study included interfacility transfer time, since patients referred from rural centres were transferred to tertiary-care centres before the initial stroke consultation.

Telestroke consultation can be performed quickly. Its efficiency compares favourably with the management of patients in rural Ontario who received tPA after being transferred from a rural hospital to a tertiary-care centre.[31] These patients had a mean total time of 138 minutes between presentation at the rural facility and drug delivery at the tertiary-care centre. Our door-to-bolus time was 106 minutes, only 36 minutes longer than that measured by the urban acute stroke service in Houston.[6] Whereas the telestroke door-to-consultation time may decrease with training and practice, interfacility transfer times, such as those observed in Ontario, are not reduced easily.

Patterns of referral

One of our referring hospitals used our telestroke service much more than the other, despite being a smaller hospital. This differential rate of referral was also found in a study of telemedicine for 657 consecutive patients at the University of California, Davis.[32] Similarly, the TESS project reported that the frequency of teleconsultation in patients with suspected stroke varied from 2% to 86% among the seven affiliated community hospitals. Possible reasons for this variation include the additional time needed for transporting the patient to the videoconference room, obtaining the patient's consent, documentation problems, lack of additional medical staff in the local hospitals, different attitudes towards thrombolysis itself as an effective treatment for acute ischaemic stroke, and underlying variation in how different physicians and facilities react to change.

User satisfaction

Videoconferencing in real-time clinical practice has yielded high levels of patient and physician satisfaction in most specialties. A study of telemedicine-based neurology reported high levels of physician and patient satisfaction for technical aspects, process and effectiveness.[33] In the TESS project, patients were satisfied with the telemedicine-based examination and commented that it was easy to speak to and cooperate with the remote neurologist. The imaging quality of both patients and CT images was considered good by the stroke neurologists. The audio quality, however, was rated mediocre, especially by the physician on the scene.

Our unpublished satisfaction data also show excellent patient and physician satisfaction following each of 26 telestroke consultations. We rated satisfaction on a Likert scale (1, agree; 2, neutral; 3, disagree) with statements based on those developed by Craig and colleagues[33] that related to technical quality, process and efficacy. Full results are shown in Fig. 6.3. Patients felt confident in the quality of a neurological evaluation performed from a distance and felt that this consultation added value over what would have been available locally. Many expressed the view that it was as good as a face-to-face encounter, suggesting that high-quality videoconferencing does not disrupt the patient–doctor interaction, even in the setting of urgent care.

Subacute care and management

In other experiences, subacute telestroke consultation has been shown to improve resource allocation in post-stroke management by reducing the length of hospital stay.

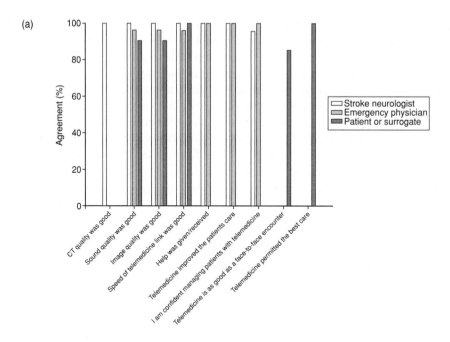

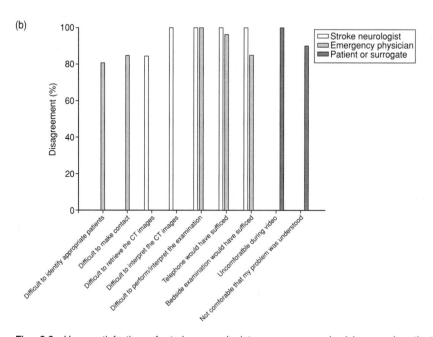

Fig. 6.3. User satisfaction of stroke neurologists, emergency physicians and patients or surrogates, shown as the percentage of each group noting (a) agreement with positive statements and (b) disagreement with negative statements.

CT, computed tomography.

In one of two small rural hospitals in Ireland, patients were offered a neurological consultation with a neurologist situated 120 km away using a real-time videolink. Hospital stay was significantly shorter for those admitted to the hospital with telemedicine resources ($p < 0.05$). Diagnosis by the teleneurologist was accurate in all cases, although there was no difference in overall mortality between the groups.[34]

In addition to access to thrombolysis, referral to stroke centres may also be important for the comprehensive quality of care in all patients presenting to hospital with stroke.[35] A study of patterns of care among patients with suspected stroke presenting to emergency departments in rural east Texas hospitals revealed that head CT scanning and ECG monitoring were performed in only 88% and 85% of patients, respectively, and blood-pressure lowering was inappropriately aggressive, yielding pressures below current recommendations.[5] Other studies have shown that telephone consultation for cognitive testing may provide a useful method for the diagnosis of post-stroke dementia.[36] Even after discharge, telemedicine-enabled family discussions may be helpful for caregivers of stroke survivors.[37] In addition, telemedicine is useful for stroke rehabilitation in the subacute or post-discharge setting.[38]

Networks of care

In a recent US survey by the Brain Attack Coalition (BAC), less than 10% of hospitals met criteria for a primary stroke centre despite the fact that over 75% of responding neurologists, neurosurgeons and emergency physicians felt that their own hospital did. The BAC has offered consensus guidelines for criteria for a hospital to be designated as a primary stroke centre, including acute stroke teams, stroke units, written care protocols, an integrated emergency response system, around-the-clock availability and interpretation of CT, and rapid laboratory testing.[3] One community hospital in suburban Maryland has implemented such guidelines and has increased successfully the proportion of patients treated safely with IV tPA.[39] Participation in a telestroke network may permit a community hospital to meet these guidelines, thereby increasing the delivery of appropriate therapies and reducing peri-stroke complications without the costly addition of equipment or personnel.

Future technologies

Improvements in videoconferencing should increase the quality of the received picture, improving the accuracy of interpreting clinical signs. In addition, mobile or wireless telemedicine may permit earlier diagnosis and management by allowing an interview and clinical examination of a patient in the field or during transportation by paramedics in an ambulance. A recent case report has documented the first delivery of tPA by a non-physician healthcare worker at a hospital in rural Texas networked by a telestroke system to a stroke centre in Houston.[40]

Conclusion

In neurologically underserved communities and in rural settings, thrombolysis remains a therapy of limited availability. Telemedicine consultation permits a reliable acute stroke evaluation in real time using videoconferencing and the transmission of non-contrast CT images. These systems not only promote increased rates of tPA use in appropriately selected patients but also improve the quality of subacute care. The participation of the community hospital is pivotal for successful referral. Evaluation of patients in the community setting prevents the use of expensive transport before diagnosis and optimizes the use of scarce resources. Despite requiring changes in workflow and patient–doctor dynamics, telestroke consultation yields high levels of satisfaction from both clinicians and patients. Furthermore, the technology provides a useful method of establishing primary stroke centres and stroke networks of care for clinical and research applications. Additional prospective controlled trials should confirm these findings in larger networks of care.

References

1 American Heart Association. *Heart Disease and Stroke Statistics: 2003 Update*. Dallas, TX: American Heart Association, 2002.
2 Tissue plasminogen activator for acute ischemic stroke. The National Institute of Neurological Disorders and Stroke rt-PA Stroke Study Group. *New England Journal of Medicine* 1995; **333**: 1581–1587.
3 Alberts MJ, Hademenos G, Latchaw RE *et al*. Recommendations for the establishment of primary stroke centers. Brain Attack Coalition. *Journal of the American Medical Association* 2000; **283**: 3102–3109.
4 Lacy CR, Suh DC, Bueno M, Kostis JB. Delay in presentation and evaluation for acute stroke: Stroke Time Registry for Outcomes Knowledge and Epidemiology (S.T.R.O.K.E.). *Stroke* 2001; **32**: 63–69.
5 Burgin WS, Staub L, Chan W *et al*. Acute stroke care in non-urban emergency departments. *Neurology* 2001; **57**: 2006–2012.
6 Grotta JC, Burgin WS, El-Mitwalli A *et al*. Intravenous tissue-type plasminogen activator therapy for ischemic stroke: Houston experience 1996 to 2000. *Archives of Neurology* 2001; **58**: 2009–2013.
7 Katzan IL, Furlan AJ, Lloyd LE *et al*. Use of tissue-type plasminogen activator for acute ischemic stroke: the Cleveland area experience. *Journal of the American Medical Association* 2000; **283**: 1151–1158.
8 Katzan IL, Hammer MD, Furlan AJ *et al*. Quality improvement and tissue-type plasminogen activator for acute ischemic stroke: a Cleveland update. *Stroke* 2003; **34**: 799–800.
9 Hanson SK, Brauer DJ, Anderson DC *et al*. Stroke Treatment in the Community (STIC): intravenous rt-PA in clinical practice. *Neurology* 1998; **50**: A155–A156.
10 Bravata DM, Kim N, Concato J *et al*. Thrombolysis for acute stroke in routine clinical practice. *Archives of Internal Medicine* 2002; **162**: 1994–2001.
11 Silliman SL, Quinn B, Huggett V, Merino JG. Use of a field-to-stroke center helicopter transport program to extend thrombolytic therapy to rural residents. *Stroke* 2003; **34**: 729–733.
12 Mavrogeni SI, Tsirintani M, Kleanthous C *et al*. Supervision of thrombolysis of acute myocardial infarction using telemedicine. *Journal of Telemedicine and Telecare* 2000; **6**: 54–58.
13 Pysher L, Harlow C. Teleradiology using low-cost consumer-oriented computer hardware and software. *American Journal of Roentgenology* 1999; **172**: 1181–1184.
14 Apple SL, Schmidt JH. Technique for neurosurgically relevant CT image transfers using inexpensive video digital technology. *Surgery and Neurology* 2000; **53**: 411–416.
15 Levine SR, Gorman M. 'Telestroke': the application of telemedicine for stroke. *Stroke* 1999; **30**: 464–469.
16 Craig JJ, McConville JP, Patterson VH, Wootton R. Neurological examination is possible using telemedicine. *Journal of Telemedicine and Telecare* 1999; **5**: 177–181.
17 Shafqat S, Kvedar JC, Guanci MM *et al*. Role for telemedicine in acute stroke: feasibility and reliability of remote administration of the NIH Stroke Scale. *Stroke* 1999; **30**: 2141–2145.
18 Goldstein LB, Bertels C, Davis JN. Interrater reliability of the NIH Stroke Scale. *Archives of Neurology* 1989; **46**: 660–662.
19 Wang S, Lee SB, Pardue C *et al*. Remote evaluation of acute ischemic stroke: reliability of National Institutes of Health Stroke Scale via telestroke. *Stroke* 2003; **34**: e188–e191.
20 Handschu R, Littmann R, Reulbach U *et al*. Telemedicine in emergency evaluation of acute stroke: interrater agreement in remote video examination with a novel multimedia system. *Stroke* 2003; **34**: 2842–2846.

21   Von Kummer R, Allen KL, Holle R *et al.* Acute stroke: usefulness of early CT findings before thrombolytic therapy. *Radiology* 1997; **205**: 327–333.

22   Hacke W, Kaste M, Fieschi C *et al.* Intravenous thrombolysis with recombinant tissue plasminogen activator for acute hemispheric stroke. The European Cooperative Acute Stroke Study (ECASS). *Journal of the American Medical Association* 1995; **274**: 1017–1025.

23   Buchan AM, Barber PA, Newcommon N *et al.* Effectiveness of t-PA in acute ischemic stroke: outcome relates to appropriateness. *Neurology* 2000; **54**: 679–684.

24   Kalafut MA, Schriger DL, Saver JL, Starkman S. Detection of early CT signs of > 1/3 middle cerebral artery infarctions: interrater reliability and sensitivity of CT interpretation by physicians involved in acute stroke care. *Stroke* 2000; **31**: 1667–1671.

25   Johnston KC, Worrall BB. Teleradiology Assessment of Computerized Tomographs Online Reliability Study (TRACTORS) for acute stroke evaluation. *Telemedicine Journal and e-Health* 2003; **9**: 227–233.

26   Schwamm LH, Rosenthal ES, Hirshberg A *et al.* Virtual TeleStroke support for the emergency department evaluation of acute stroke. *Academic Emergency Medicine* 2004; **11**: 1193–1197.

27   Clark WM, Wissman S, Albers GW *et al.* Recombinant tissue-type plasminogen activator (Alteplase) for ischemic stroke 3 to 5 hours after symptom onset. The ATLANTIS Study: a randomized controlled trial. Alteplase Thrombolysis for Acute Noninterventional Therapy in Ischemic Stroke. *Journal of the American Medical Association* 1999; **282**: 2019–2026.

28   Wiborg A, Widder B. Teleneurology to improve stroke care in rural areas: the Telemedicine in Stroke in Swabia (TESS) Project. *Stroke* 2003; **34**: 2951–2956.

29   Wang S, Gross H, Lee SB *et al.* Remote evaluation of acute ischemic stroke in rural community hospitals in Georgia. *Stroke* 2004; **35**: 1763–1768.

30   Audebert HJ, Kukla C, Clarmann von Claranau S *et al.* Telemedicine for safe and extended use of thrombolysis in stroke. The Telemedic Pilot Project for Integrative Stroke Care (TEMPiS) in Bavaria. *Stroke* 2005; **36**; 287–291.

31   Merino JG, Silver B, Wong E *et al.* Extending tissue plasminogen activator use to community and rural stroke patients. *Stroke* 2002; **33**: 141–146.

32   Nesbitt TS, Hilty DM, Kuenneth CA, Siefkin A. Development of a telemedicine program: a review of 1,000 videoconferencing consultations. *Western Journal of Medicine* 2000; **173**: 169–174.

33   Craig J, Russell C, Patterson V, Wootton R. User satisfaction with realtime teleneurology. *Journal of Telemedicine and Telecare* 1999; **5**: 237–241.

34   Craig J, Chua R, Russell C *et al.* A cohort study of early neurological consultation by telemedicine on the care of neurological inpatients. *Journal of Neurology, Neurosurgery and Psychiatry* 2004; **75**: 1031–1035.

35   Crome O, Bahr M. Editorial comment – remote evaluation of acute ischemic stroke: a reliable tool to extend tissue plasminogen activator use to community and rural stroke patients? *Stroke* 2003; **34**: e191–e192.

36   Barber M, Stott DJ. Validity of the Telephone Interview for Cognitive Status (TICS) in post-stroke subjects. *International Journal of Geriatric Psychiatry* 2004; **19**: 75–79.

37   Grant JS, Elliott TR, Weaver M *et al.* Telephone intervention with family caregivers of stroke survivors after rehabilitation. *Stroke* 2002; **33**: 2060–2065.

38   Holden MK, Dyar T, Schwamm L, Bizzi E. Home-based telerehabilitation using a virtual environment system. In: *Proceedings of the 2nd International Workshop on Virtual Rehabilitation.* Burdea GC, Thalmann D, Lewis JA, eds. Piscataway, NJ 2003; pp. 4–12.

39   Lattimore SU, Chalela J, Davis L *et al.* Impact of establishing a primary stroke center at a community hospital on the use of thrombolytic therapy: the NINDS Suburban Hospital Stroke Center experience. *Stroke* 2003; **34**: e55–e57.

40   Choi JY, Wojner AW, Cale RT *et al.* Telemedicine physician providers: augmented acute stroke care delivery in rural Texas: an initial experience. *Telemedicine Journal and e-Health* 2004; **10**: S90–S94.

7

Telemedicine in Rehabilitation

Elsie Hui

Introduction

Telerehabilitation is the assessment, diagnosis, direct therapy, education, monitoring and support of patients at remote sites via telecommunication methods, ranging from use of the telephone to videoconferencing through the Internet or dedicated digital links. Rudimentary telerehabilitation was developed to provide care to disabled patients living in remote areas, who, due to their physical limitations, had particular difficulty in travelling to urban rehabilitation facilities. Since then, significant advances have been made in the technology involved, both in the equipment used to provide direct patient care and in the stations and networks used to link therapist and patient. It has been suggested that telerehabilitation could become an important modality to service providers who are seeking to extend post-acute care into a non-clinical setting.[1] For example, by extending rehabilitation beyond the hospital and into the community or into the home, providers can continue to monitor patients' progress, identify areas in need of improvement before complications set in, and ultimately improve patient function and decrease long-term disability and costs.[2]

Overview

While many centres are using telemedicine to provide otherwise conventional rehabilitative care to patients with neurological diseases, some researchers are exploring the use of human–computer interface systems to enhance the quality of care provided and, hence, clinical outcomes.[3-5] With the increasing availability and affordability of home computers and Internet connections, the cost of telerehabilitation has fallen substantially in recent years. Telerehabilitation has been applied in numerous neurological conditions, including stroke, brain and spinal injury, and cognitive impairment. In addition to direct links between patients and healthcare professionals, disease-specific websites provide important information on neurological conditions to patients and their families and carers.

Home-based teletherapy

Home-based teletherapy is the delivery of healthcare, in particular physical therapy, to disabled patients at home. Researchers at the Jim Thorpe Rehabilitation Center in

Oklahoma, USA, described a 52-year-old stroke patient receiving telerehabilitation using an ordinary telephone system.[6] The patient and the therapist were connected via a desktop videophone transmitting at a maximum speed of 33.6 kbit/s. (For comparison, videoconferencing in telemedicine commonly uses bandwidths 10 times higher than this to achieve better-quality video pictures.) Over 17 months, the patient received physical therapy, speech therapy, psychological support and vocational rehabilitation from a team of rehabilitation specialists. Improvements in physical, functional and psychological outcomes were observed.

The audio and video quality of earlier systems was poor, with frequent interruptions during the sessions. Nevertheless, such systems improved the access to care in severely handicapped people residing in remote locations.

Commercial videoconferencing equipment is extremely effective in the delivery of telerehabilitation consultations for cases with neurological conditions. Although the high cost of these systems precludes their use in the homes of individuals, they have been introduced in rural clinics, nursing homes and schools. Specialist clinicians from urban centres can work with physicians, nurses, teachers and other caregivers in remote settings, augmenting the level of care and minimizing the number of trips that need to be made by both the specialist and the patient.[7,8] This system is well established in vast countries such as Australia and the USA.

Human–computer interface systems in stroke rehabilitation

Multidisciplinary rehabilitation has been shown to improve functional outcomes and reduce mortality following stroke.[9] More intensive speech and language therapy was found to produce significant improvements in language.[10] In motor recovery, task-specific approaches that deal with lost abilities are superior to more traditional treatments, such as repetitive training and resistance exercises.[11] The use of robotics and virtual reality as an adjunct to traditional stroke therapy provided by human professionals has been studied. Volpe and colleagues developed a robotic device that interacted with the patient in real time by measuring a patient's upper-limb movement and, if necessary, guided the arm through a stereotyped pattern.[12] By allowing subjects to re-learn shoulder and elbow coordination, robot-assisted sensorimotor training produced significantly improved motor function of the upper limb as well as overall functional outcome (Functional Independence Measurement – Motor). Moreover, the use of robotic devices allows the physical therapist to focus on more task-specific and complex functional movements.

Virtual reality is a computer technology that simulates real-life tasks. By attaching sensors to the patient's body, the computer can measure, evaluate and provide feedback to the patient in real time. Virtual environments can improve patient motivation by providing a more engaging interface to the exercises. Burdea's group at Rutgers University has developed a game-like virtual reality exercise system for both the upper and the lower limb. These are designed to motivate and challenge the patient to work harder, by providing information on their performance.[13]

By integrating the above virtual reality-based rehabilitation system with robotics, in this case a haptic glove (Fig. 7.1), a web-based telerehabilitation monitoring system was produced. Data on the patient's performance are sent in real time to a remote therapist and displayed as a three-dimensional mock-up of the relevant body part (eg the hand) on the therapist's computer screen (Fig. 7.2). Virtual reality using Java3D simulates the patient's movements. The therapist can communicate instantaneously with the patient via a microphone and make modifications to the exercise routine. Data can also be transferred periodically to a server for storage. Using the web portal, the therapist can see a patient's progress over time, in the form of performance timeline

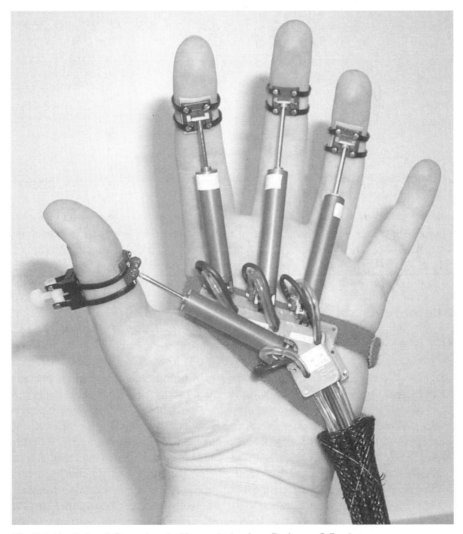

Fig. 7.1. Haptic hand. Reproduced with permission from Professor G Burdea.

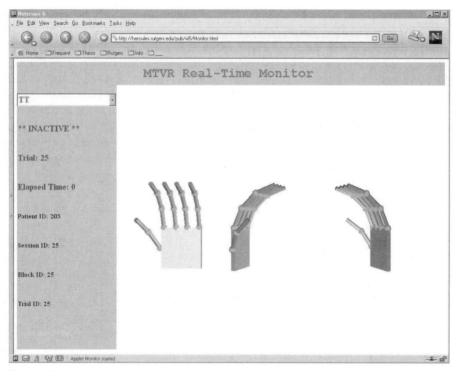

Fig. 7.2. Physiotherapist's screen.

graphs. This technology allows a patient more therapy time in their own home, and increases the number of patients that a healthcare professional can monitor and help at any one time.[14]

Internet-based cognitive rehabilitation

One example of Internet-based telerehabilitation is the website NeuroPsychOnline (NPO) (www.neuropsychonline.com/) (Fig. 7.3). This focuses on neuropsychological diagnosis and cognitive rehabilitation, with patient groups ranging from children with learning and developmental disabilities[15] to adults recovering from brain injury[16]. A commercially available multimedia program, Psychological Software Services (www.neuroscience.cnter.com/pss/PSSCogRehab/moreinfo.htm), is offered to healthcare facilities and professionals via a membership scheme, so that they in turn can offer telerehabilitation to their patients. The whole system, including applications and data, can be delivered over the Internet. The cognitive rehabilitation system of NPO has 50 online exercises focusing on attention, execution, memory, visuospatial, problem-solving and communication skills. The software continuously monitors the patient's performance, and the skill level can be adjusted either automatically by the program or manually by the therapist. The beauty of the system is that patients can

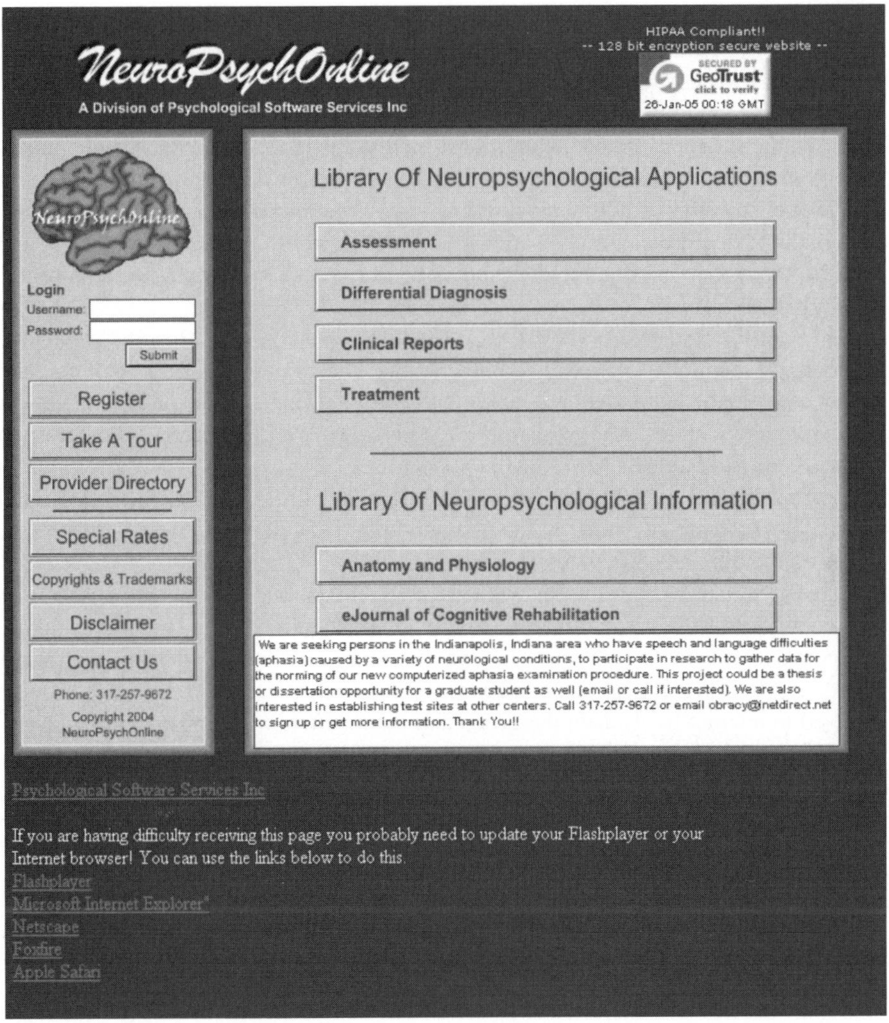

Fig. 7.3. NeuroPsychOnline web page.

access telerehabilitation from any computer connected to the Internet and continue their therapy at home and elsewhere. Clinicians can monitor patients' progress through progress reports, and pooled data from the central database at NPO also provide useful information to individual subscribers.

Telerehabilitation in Hong Kong

In Hong Kong, telemedicine was introduced in the late 1990s, with applications in various medical specialties (see http://tele.med.cuhk.edu.hk/index.htm). Initially, we established a network to support local nursing homes,[8] but we recognized the unmet needs of senior citizens with chronic diseases who were residing in the community. A study was launched in 2003 to study the feasibility and efficacy of delivering rehabilitation programmes by videoconferencing to small groups of older patients with common chronic medical conditions, such as diabetes, knee pain, dementia and urinary incontinence, as well as stroke. Telerehabilitation was considered an attractive alternative to more traditional hospital- or clinic-based programmes, because potentially it could reach more patients and make use of community resources and because the 'group' model may have advantages over conventional one-to-one care-delivery models.

Three teleconferencing sites were established: at Shatin Hospital and two community centres for senior citizens in the same district. Commercial videoconferencing equipment was used (at the hospital site, a model 880, Tandberg; at the community centres, a ViewStation FX, Polycom). We used Internet Protocol (IP) transmission over a dedicated 10-Mbit/s local-area network (LAN) and were able to support multipoint transmission. Dual video outputs allowed the subjects to see the instructor (a research assistant with nursing or allied health training) and PowerPoint slides on two separate 86-cm television screens.

Subjects either were referred by their physician or were members of a church community centre. They had the relevant clinical diagnosis and were able to follow on-screen instructions. Each programme consisted of three components: physical exercise or training, education and peer-group support. At each session, subjects were allowed to interact freely with the group and the instructor. Discussion among group members was encouraged. Significantly improved outcome measures were observed in the diabetes and knee-pain groups whereas in the dementia and urinary incontinence groups, videoconferencing was as effective as face-to-face rehabilitation. The stroke telerehabilitation programme[17] is of particular relevance to this book and is described in greater detail below.

Telerehabilitation: a new model for community-based stroke rehabilitation

Studies have found community-based stroke rehabilitation to be cost-effective,[18] and significant improvement in the mobility level of stroke patients can be achieved.[19] Community-based stroke rehabilitation in Hong Kong is, however, relatively underdeveloped, and current services lack psychosocial support, are utilized poorly due to transportation problems, and have inadequate collaboration between hospital and community service providers. In addition, costly inpatient rehabilitation is a very significant socioeconomic burden, and there is pressure to discharge stroke cases earlier. Thus, there is a need for a convenient, easily accessible and cost-effective model of community-based stroke rehabilitation.

There are several advantages of using telemedicine in community-based rehabilitation. First, it allows participants to access the service more readily if videoconference systems can be installed at community centres near their homes.

Second, therapy conducted as a group may enhance the atmosphere for learning. Third, it allows real-time interaction between participants and healthcare professionals. Multi-site links can increase the number of participants at any one time. However, because traditional stroke rehabilitation has always been conducted face to face, the feasibility, efficacy and acceptability of telerehabilitation in stroke patients needed to be shown. To do this, we used the setup referred to above.

Subjects had a history of stroke for at least six months and were able to walk independently, with or without walking aids. Patients with cognitive impairment, communication difficulties and severe cardiorespiratory problems were excluded. Subjects undertook an eight-week intervention programme (one session per week, comprising 1.5 hours per session) conducted by a physical therapist via a videoconference link (hardware described above). The class size was about six to eight subjects. A non-professional assistant was stationed at the community centre to facilitate the smooth running of the programme. The intervention consisted of education, exercise and social support. The education component included talks covering the pathophysiology of stroke, signs and symptoms, medical management, rehabilitation pathways, risk-factor identification, modification, psychosocial impact, community support, and home and environmental safety.

The exercise programme was designed to improve strength and balance (Fig. 7.4). The participants were encouraged to do the same exercises at home at least three times

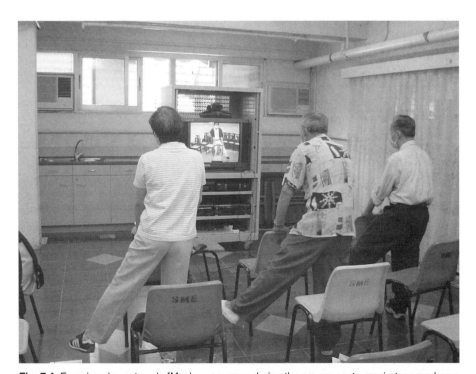

Fig. 7.4. Exercise class at work. [Masks were worn during the severe acute respiratory syndrome (SARS) epidemic in Hong Kong.]

a week, prompted by an exercise logbook. The outcome measures were the Berg Balance Scale (BBS),[20] the Medical Outcomes Study Short Form (SF-36),[21] the State Self-Esteem Scale (SSES)[22] and the Stroke Knowledge Test.[23] Satisfaction was measured by a structured questionnaire supplemented by focus groups. Twenty-one subjects were recruited in six months, but only 19 completed the eight-week intervention. Significant improvement was observed in the BBS, SSES, Stroke Knowledge Test and all subscales of SF-36 compared with baseline (Table 7.1). All eight baseline subscales scores of SF-36 in this study were lower than the age-equivalent population norms.[24] Following intervention, the subjects showed similar

Table 7.1. Pre- and post-intervention scores of four primary outcomes: the Berg Balance Scale (BBS), State Self-Esteem Scale (SSES), Medical Outcomes Study Short Form (SF-36) and Stroke Knowledge Test were compared using a paired t-test ($n = 19$)

	Pre-intervention mean (SD)	Post-intervention mean (SD)	Population-based mean
BBS	42.2 (6.7)	49.0 (6.5)[a]	NA
SSES	64.8 (12.3)	79.8 (12.8)[a]	NA
SF-36			
Physical functioning	49.0 (15.7)	71.6 (21.7)[a]	79.2 (19.7)
Role physical	18.4 (32.1)	79.0 (41.9)[a]	73.7 (37.2)
Bodily pain	57.4 (29.3)	86.0 (24.3)[a]	77.4 (26.7)
General health	35.0 (20.3)	53.2 (17.7)[a]	49.2 (21.2)
Vitality	40.8 (16.3)	66.3 (17.7)[a]	59.9 (19.8)
Social functioning	68.4 (22.2)	88.8 (19.5)[a]	92.1 (17.3)
Role emotional	45.6 (38.8)	93.0 (23.8)[a]	78.1 (37.2)
Mental health	65.3 (22.2)	77.7 (17.4)[b]	75.7 (18.1)
Stroke Knowledge Test	4.8 (1.7)	8.7 (1.5)[a]	NA

Compared with baseline values: [a]$p < 0.001$; [b]$p < 0.05$.
NA, not available; SD, standard deviation

trends or even higher subscale scores compared with the population norms.

Regarding satisfaction and feedback from the subjects, 63% and 37% rated the clinical effectiveness of telerehabilitation as good and excellent, respectively. All subjects rated the visual and audio quality as good. They expressed no preference for telerehabilitation or face-to-face treatment. All subjects accepted the use of videoconferencing for delivery of the intervention. During the meeting of the focus group, most subjects felt that the programme had been very useful. Education helped to decrease their fear of recurrent stroke (Fig. 7.5). They also felt that the programme provided for continuation of their rehabilitation. Some felt that it had psychosocial benefits for them.

The baseline data showed that the subjects had poor psychosocial status following rehabilitation in the acute phase of stroke, even though most survivors were able to function at a reasonable level. The mean initial score on the BBS was 42.2, indicating a high risk of falling. More than half of the subjects had symptoms of depression. The

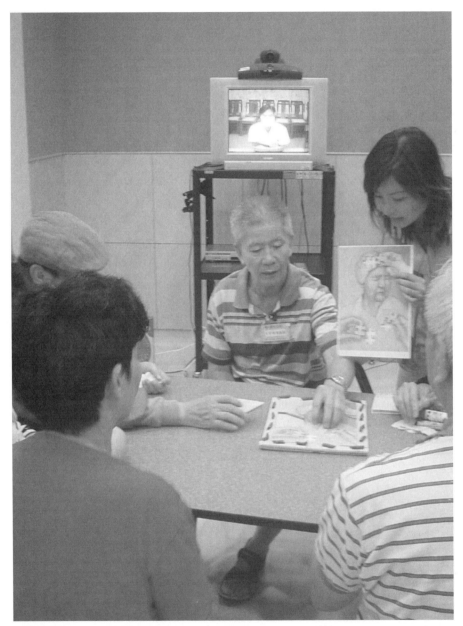

Fig. 7.5. Stroke education in progress. The therapist is on the screen and a helper is facilitating the class.

baseline subscales scores of SF-36 in the subjects were lower than the population norms. Nonetheless, the study demonstrated successfully the feasibility, efficacy and acceptability of telerehabilitation in stroke patients living in the community. It improved both physical functioning and psychosocial wellbeing in the subjects. It also demonstrated that collaboration between the hospital and community sectors was able to fill an important service gap for a potentially large population of people. Further studies with larger sample size and multi-site application, and clients with different disease staging and functional level need to be performed.

Conclusion

Telerehabilitation is an effective means of providing services to patients without a need for both the patient and the professional to be in the same location at the same time. It has a major role in providing remote rehabilitation to patients with neurological conditions. New technologies will enhance the quality and intensity of therapy delivered to the patient at home and will provide important clinical information to healthcare providers. Telerehabilitation is emerging as an alternative and possibly a more effective delivery system for rehabilitation services and shows great promise for improving patient outcomes as well as cost-savings in the near future.

Further information

Center for Advanced Information Processing, Rutger's University, Piscataway, NJ, USA. Virtual Reality/Virtual Rehabilitation Laboratory (VRLAB) Human–Machine Interface Laboratory: www.caip.rutgers.edu/aboutus/vrlab.html. Accessed 25 January 2005.

Jim Thorpe Rehabilitation Center, Oklahoma City, OK, USA. Telehealth Services Program. www.integris-health.com/INTEGRIS/en-US/Locations/okc/SMC-okc/teleheath.htm. Accessed 23 February 2005.

References

1   Palsbo SE, Bauer D. Telerehabilitation: managed care's new opportunity. *Managed Care Quarterly* 2000; **8**: 56–64.
2   Ricker JH, Rosenthal M, Garay E *et al.* Telerehabilitation needs: a survey of persons with acquired brain injury. *Journal of Head Trauma Rehabilitation* 2002; **17**: 242–250.
3   Piron L, Tonin P, Atzori AM *et al.* Virtual environment system for motor tele-rehabilitation. *Studies in Health Technology and Informatics* 2002; **85**: 355–361.
4   Rydmark M, Broeren J, Pascher R. Stroke rehabilitation at home using virtual reality, haptics and telemedicine. *Studies in Health Technology and Informatics* 2002; **85**: 434–437.
5   Rizzo AA, Strickland D, Bouchard S. The challenge of using virtual reality in telerehabilitation. *Telemedicine Journal and e-Health* 2004; **10**: 184–195.
6   Clark PG, Dawson SJ, Scheideman-Miller C, Post ML. TeleRehab: stroke teletherapy and management using two-way interactive video. *Neurology Report* 2002; **26**: 87–93.
7   Savard L, Borstad A, Tkachuck J *et al.* Telerehabilitation consultations for clients with neurologic diagnoses: cases from rural Minnesota and American Samoa. *NeuroRehabilitation* 2003; **18**: 93–102.
8   Hui E, Woo J. Telehealth for older patients: the Hong Kong experience. *Journal of Telemedicine and Telecare* 2002; **8** (suppl. 3): 39–41.

9   Gresham GE, Granger CV, Linn RT, Kulas MA. Status of functional outcomes for stroke survivors. *Physical Medical and Rehabilitation Clinics of North America* 1999; **10**: 957–966.

10   Bhogal SK, Teasell R, Speechley M. Intensity of aphasia therapy, impact on recovery. *Stroke* 2003; **34**: 987–993.

11   Papathanasiou I, Filipovic SR, Whurr R, Jahanshahi M. Plasticity of motor cortex excitability induced by rehabilitation therapy for writing. *Neurology* 2003; **61**: 977–980.

12   Volpe BT, Krebs HI, Hogan N. Robot-aided sensorimotor training in stroke rehabilitation. *Advances in Neurology* 2003; **92**: 429–433.

13   Merians AS, Jack D, Boian R *et al*. Virtual reality: augmented rehabilitation for patients following stroke. *Physical Therapy* 2002; **82**: 898–915.

14   Lewis J, Boian R, Burdea G, Deutsch J. Real-time web-based telerehabilitation monitoring. *Studies in Health Technology and Informatics* 2003; **94**: 190–192.

15   Bracy OL, Oakes AL, Cooper RS *et al*. The effects of cognitive rehabilitation therapy techniques for enhancing the cognitive/intellectual functioning of seventh and eighth grade children. *Cognitive Technology Journal* 1999; **4**: 19–27.

16   Chen SH, Thomas JD, Glueckauf RL, Bracy OL. The effectiveness of computer-assisted cognitive rehabilitation for persons with traumatic brain injury. *Brain Injury* 1997; **11**: 197–209.

17   Lai JC, Woo J, Hui E, Chan WM. Telerehabilitation: a new model for community-based stroke rehabilitation. *Journal of Telemedicine and Telecare* 2004; **10**: 199–205.

18   Beech R, Rudd AG, Tilling K, Wolfe CD. Economic consequences of early inpatient discharge to community-based rehabilitation for stroke in an inner-London teaching hospital. *Stroke* 1999; **30**: 729–735.

19   Phua HS. A descriptive report on the outcome of the Community Rehabilitation Program. *Physiotherapy Singapore* 2002; **5**: 4–10.

20   Berg KO, Wood-Dauphinee SL, Williams JI, Maki B. Measuring balance in the elderly: validation of an instrument. *Canadian Journal of Public Health* 1992; **83** (suppl. 2): 7–11.

21   Ware JE, Sherbourne CD. The MOS 36-item short form health survey (SF-36), I. Conceptual framework and item selection. *Medical Care* 1992; **30**: 473–483.

22   Heatherton TF, Polivy J. Development and validation of a scale for measuring state self-esteem. *Journal of Personality and Social Psychology* 1991; **60**: 895–910.

23   Kothari R, Sauerbeck L, Jauch E *et al*. Patients' awareness of stroke signs, symptoms and risks factors. *Stroke* 1997; **28**: 1871–1875.

24   Lam LK, Lauder IJ, Lam TP, Gaudek B. Population based norming of the Chinese (HK) version of the SF-36 health survey. *Hong Kong Practitioner* 1999; **21**: 460–470.

▶8

Telemedicine and Neuroradiology

Liam Caffery and Alan Coulthard

Introduction

'Teleradiology' is an umbrella term for the transfer of radiological images over a telecommunication network from one location to another. The transfer of images is computer-assisted, and in its simplest form teleradiology is two computers linked together by a network that can transmit and receive images. Teleradiology may use a local-area network (LAN) to transfer images from one part of a hospital to another or a wide-area network (WAN) to transfer images between hospitals or internationally. Neuroimaging, in particular computed tomography (CT) scanning and magnetic resonance imaging (MRI), is essential for the practice of modern neurology. Teleradiology is the means of delivering these images to a clinician who is remote from the patient. Teleradiology can be applied to neuroradiology in the same way as to the other radiological subspecialties.

History

An early example of teleradiological transfer was performed in Canada in 1959 when Dr Albert Jutras from Montreal undertook remote diagnosis of fluoroscopy images via interactive television.[1] CT was invented in the 1970s, and the first clinical scanners were installed between 1974 and 1976. CT became widely available in the 1980s, and MRI was in widespread clinical use by 1990. This was the catalyst for the development of the Digital Imaging and Communication in Medicine (DICOM) standard for digital image transfer between devices. The American College of Radiology (ACR) and the National Electrical Manufacturers Association (NEMA) first published this in 1985 after two years of development. The DICOM standard at the time of writing, version 3.0, uses the Transmission Control Protocol/Internet Protocol (TCP/IP), the networking protocol that runs the World Wide Web (WWW). This has allowed radiological devices and modalities to be connected at a distance through a network rather than by point-to-point cabling and has accelerated the development of teleradiology. Teleradiology is a mature technique embedded in everyday radiological practice.

The digital image

Radiological images must be in a digital format before they can be transmitted by a teleradiology system. A digital image is made up of a matrix of pixels or picture elements. Each of the pixels represents one homogeneous shade of grey. A digital image with 512 rows and 512 columns of pixels is said to have a 512×512-image matrix. The matrix of pixels also has depth: this is the number of shades of grey that each pixel can represent. The depth is measured in bits, eg an 8-bit image is 256 (2^8) shades of grey and an image with 4096 shades of grey is a 14-bit image. A 512×512 matrix is the standard matrix size for CT, magnetic resonance (MR) and ultrasound images. Computed radiography (CR) is a means of acquiring plain X-rays (such as chest films) in a digital format and has a matrix size of 2048×2048 pixels.

The quality of an image is governed by its spatial resolution and contrast resolution. Digital image quality is improved by increasing the matrix size (effectively reducing the pixel size), which is termed 'increasing the spatial resolution' (Fig. 8.1). Quality is also improved by increasing the bit depth of the image, which is termed 'increasing the contrast resolution' (Fig. 8.2). Because the size of an image is proportional to both the

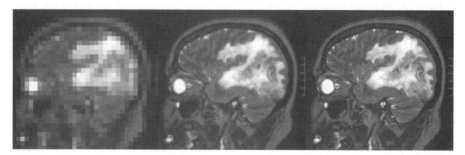

Fig. 8.1. Image quality is improved by increasing the spatial resolution.

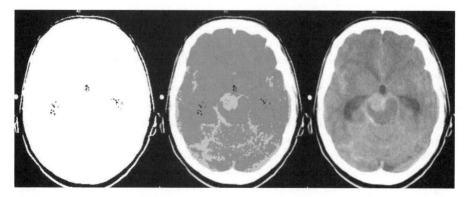

Fig. 8.2. Image quality is improved by increasing the bit depth (shown are 1-, 4- and 8-bit depths).

number of pixels in an image and the bit depth, increasing either the spatial or the contrast resolution will increase the file size of the image.

Image compression

A typical CT image will be 1 MB in size. A series of such slices may produce a dataset of 90 MB. The larger the file size, the longer it will take to transmit the file across a network. Compression techniques can be used to reduce the size of an image file, which both speeds up the transmission time (an important consideration in teleradiology networks) and reduces the storage requirements for the file. Compression is usually expressed as a ratio, eg 3:1 means that the image is compressed to one-third of its original size.

Compression can be either *lossy* or *lossless*. Lossless compression means that when the compressed image is reconstructed, the value of each pixel exactly matches the original image. When an image is compressed with lossy compression, the reconstructed image does not have exactly the same pixel value, although the image may be visually indistinguishable from the original. Lossy compression techniques yield higher compression ratios than do lossless compression techniques. Medical images can be compressed with techniques such as JPEG (Joint Photographic Experts Group) and wavelet compression.[2]

Numerous studies have shown that it is possible to compress images to a certain degree without loss of diagnostic value. Erickson[2] has found that compression ratios of 20:1 are acceptable for CT and MR images. The ACR standard for practice of teleradiology[3] allows the use of compression but does not make recommendations on the method or ratio of compression. Instead, the ACR recommends that the physician using the system is responsible for attesting that the diagnostic value of an image is not compromised when using compression.

Digital image communication

To facilitate communication between imaging devices and display workstations, an internationally agreed standard has evolved: the DICOM standard. This defines standard image formats and standard information models, such as patient demographics and protocols, for communication between devices. It also provides an open architecture, which allows the integration of medical imaging devices from different manufacturers.

A DICOM image has two parts: the header, which contains text-based information about the images and study as well as patient demographics, and the actual pixel data of the image, often in JPEG format. One of the aims of the DICOM standard is to ensure that there is no loss of image quality between image acquisition and image display. For this reason, the ACR standard for the practice of teleradiology[3] recommends the use of DICOM when implementing teleradiology. Many radiology departments are moving towards a complete networked digital imaging environment, in which images are acquired in a digital format and stored in a central database and all modalities are networked. Images are viewed by clinicians in 'soft copy' on a computer monitor. These systems are referred to as picture-archiving and communication systems (PACS). PACS also uses the DICOM standard.

Components of a teleradiology system

A teleradiology system is made up of the following components:

▶ image-acquisition modalities

▶ image server

▶ telecommunication network

▶ receiving station

▶ review station.

Image-acquisition modalities

Modalities such as CT, MR and ultrasound produce digital images. If these modalities are DICOM-compliant, then they can transfer images into a teleradiology image server using the DICOM standard. An alternative method of producing a digital image is to use a film scanner or film digitizer to convert an analogue image to digital format. To do this, a sheet of film printed with images is scanned to produce the digital image. The level of sophistication of film scanners varies, and the resultant digital image may be in DICOM format or another image format, eg JPEG or TIFF (tagged image file format). This digital image is then transferred to the teleradiology image server. A film digitizer is often the cheapest way to implement teleradiology (Fig. 8.3).

Image server

An image server, also known as a transmit server or a compression server, can store images from acquisition devices, compress them if required and transfer them to a receiving station. The transfer of images can be either by a *push* method, whereby the image server transmits images to the receiving station, or a *pull* method, whereby the receiving station requests them. Pull methodology is used when implementing web-based teleradiology systems. In such systems, the clinician using the web browser (web client) requests images from the image server by entering details, eg the patient's name.

Telecommunication network

There are many kinds of telecommunication networks, and the decision regarding which to use for a teleradiology system is based on the size of the image file, the transmission speed required for clinical need, privacy considerations and cost. The network could be either an entirely private network, such as an intranet within or between hospitals, or a public network using integrated services digital network

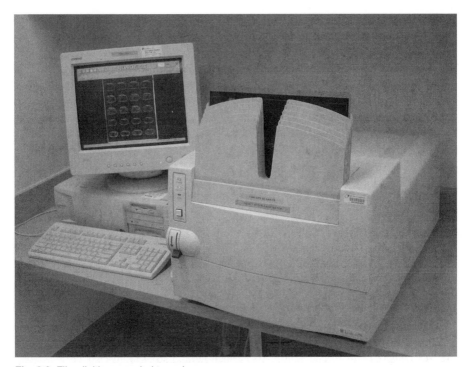

Fig. 8.3. Film digitizer coupled to an image server.

(ISDN) lines, asymmetric digital subscriber lines (ADSL) or cable Internet, available from commercial telecommunication carriers.

Receiving station

A receiving station will accept images transmitted from an image server and will then either allow the review of these images by a coupled display station or archive the images to serve multiple display stations.

Review station

A review station is typically a personal computer (PC) running image-viewing software. The software allows the user to display and manipulate the images. Image-manipulation functions include changing the brightness and contrast, zooming, panning and magnifying the image. The display station is coupled to a monitor, which may be a standard PC monitor or a high-resolution greyscale monitor suitable for primary interpretation of the images (Fig. 8.4).

Implementing teleradiology

Teleradiology can be implemented in numerous ways, which vary in image quality and cost.

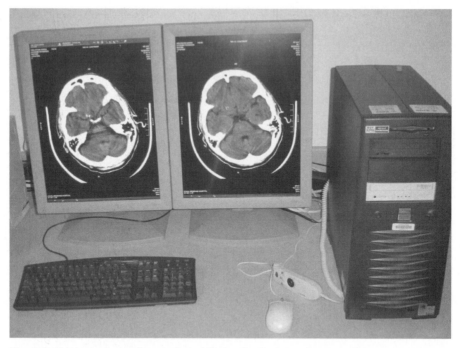

Fig. 8.4. Dual monitor review station, with image-viewing software running on a personal computer.

Dedicated teleradiology systems

Commercial teleradiology systems can be purchased from numerous vendors. These systems often consist only of an image server and receiving station, allowing the flexibility to use a telecommunication network of choice. The image file format used by the teleradiology system, whether it is DICOM or otherwise, is an important consideration in the purchase of a teleradiology system. The ACR recommends that if a written report is produced from the teleradiology images, then the DICOM standard should be used. The ACR also makes the following recommendations regarding the software and the monitors used to view images:

▶ ability to window the image's brightness and contrast

▶ ability to magnify and zoom the image

▶ ability to perform accurate measurements, such as distances and angles

▶ ability to display patient demographics on the screen with the images

▶ monitor brightness of at least 175 cd/m².

Images not intended for primary reporting can utilize non-DICOM image formats such as JPEG. There is no standard related to the monitor or software required to review images, so a standard PC monitor can be used.

Using PACS to implement teleradiology

PACS-enabled hospitals can use existing equipment to implement teleradiology in a number of ways:

▶ *Data warehousing.* A number of hospitals can archive their images to a central location, allowing images from any feeding hospital to be viewed at any of the sites.

▶ *Remote modality.* In the same way that a CT scanner in a radiology department can be networked to the PACS, a CT scanner at a remote location can be networked to the PACS over a WAN. This enables images acquired at the remote location to be archived and viewed by clinicians using the PACS.

▶ *Remote viewing station.* A viewing station can be connected to a PACS over a WAN, allowing the user to view images archived on the PACS. This technique is often used by on-call radiologists to view images at home.

▶ *PACS-to-PACS image transfer.* A PACS at one hospital can be configured to send images to a PACS located at another hospital. This technique is often used when a patient's care is transferred from one facility to another.

Web-based teleradiology

Web-based teleradiology systems can either use the full DICOM image set or a compressed image format. The main advantages of web-based teleradiology systems are that, because images are viewed using a web browser, no special teleradiology software needs to be installed on the client computer and training requirements are minimal. The main disadvantage is the lag time before the images can be viewed.

External service providers

A number of organizations have started to provide teleradiology services, including Nighthawk Teleradiology, Virtual Radiological Clinics, International Teleradiology Services, PRO Radiology and Teleradiology Consulting. All of these organizations use broadband Internet connections and web-based teleradiology systems to provide a radiology reporting service that includes neuroradiology. These groups are not affiliated with any particular hospital and may provide a teleradiology service to multiple institutions in different countries. In keeping with the recommendations from professional bodies, they rely on DICOM interfaces to transfer images from the modality to their teleradiology web server.

These services may well be less costly for client hospitals, since they need not employ a radiologist for daytime or on-call work and will not have to bear the costs of teleradiology systems of their own.

Applications

Applications of teleradiology in neurology include its use in neurosurgery and in stroke.

Neurosurgery

Neurosurgical units are usually based at hospitals in major cities that have other neuroscience specialties and facilities such as intensive care units. Traumatic brain injury and other emergency neurosurgical problems, however, often occur at some distance from these centres, and teleradiology can be used to bridge this distance. By reviewing a patient's CT scans over teleradiology links, a neurosurgeon can advise a referring doctor on whether transfer of the patient to the tertiary centre is warranted and the urgency of transfer and appropriate therapy needed before transfer. Evidence on the effectiveness of such systems has been reported from Italy,[4] South Africa,[5] France[6] and Norway.[7] In Hong Kong, teleradiology has been shown to reduce unwarranted patient transfers by 21% and to minimize adverse events, such as hypoxia and hypotension, during transfer by 24%.[8]

Interventional neuroradiology is a relatively new discipline, which, like neurosurgery, is usually based at urban tertiary referral centres. Teleradiology also has an important role here in ensuring wider geographical access, as in the following case report.

Case report 1

A 69-year-old man presented to a neurosurgeon with a six-month history of worsening right-sided cerebellar symptoms, ataxia and intermittent headache. On examination, the patient was found to have a mild weakness of the right face. A CT angiogram obtained locally showed a complex unruptured aneurysm of the distal left vertebral/proximal basilar artery (Fig. 8.5a). MRI suggested that this was partially thrombosed (Fig. 8.5b). An opinion was sought from a specialist neuroradiologist at the neurointervention centre 1350 km away. The CT and MR studies were transferred to the PACS for review by the radiologists, who determined that further staging studies were warranted before deciding on appropriate management. The patient was transferred to the neurointervention centre electively and underwent catheter angiography of the cerebral vessels with three-dimensional (3D) rotational views and computer-generated 3D imaging (Fig. 8.5c,d). On the basis of these images, it was determined that the aneurysm was potentially treatable by endovascular means. The neuroradiologist was able to discuss the case with the referring neurosurgeon, and between them a decision was made to manage the patient conservatively, as the symptoms were stable and relatively minor.

Stroke

Teleradiology in the treatment of acute stroke has been documented in a number of studies, where the use of teleradiology has been employed for review of CT scans.[9,10] If intravenous tissue plasminogen activator (IV tPA) is to be used for patients suffering

(a)

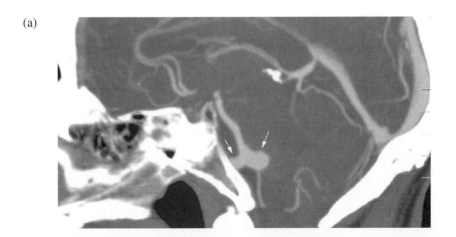

(b)

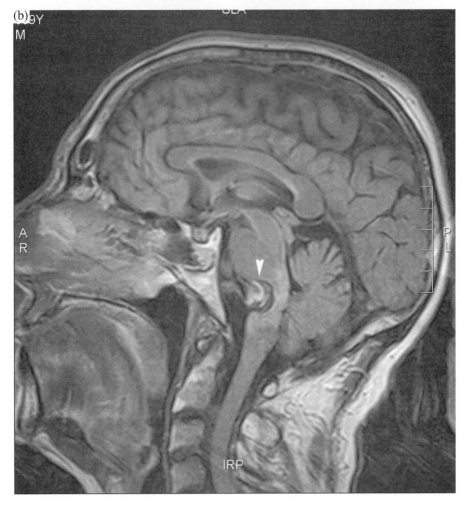

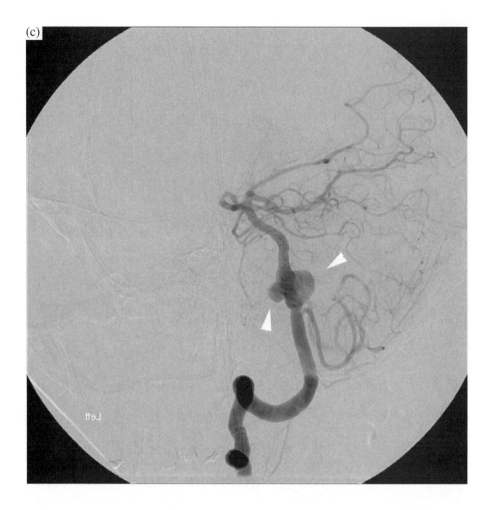

acute ischaemic stroke, then it must be administered within three hours of the onset of symptoms. Review of CT head scans for contraindications, such as haemorrhage and large infarct size, is time-critical, and teleradiology is the only way to do this at hospitals that do not have specialist neurological or neuroradiological cover. Time-savings can also be achieved by using teleradiology links to a specialist's home when cover is provided in an 'on-call' situation.

A study of emergency teleradiological review of CT scans in Austria documented the speed of teleradiology services. The majority (83%) of 422 patients with severe neurological problems had a written legal final report available to the referring clinician within one hour.[11] The Teleradiology Assessment of Computerized Tomographs Online Reliability Study (TRACTORS)[12] found that when reviewing CT scans to determine eligibility for IV tPA, a neurologist with stroke expertise could read CT scans using teleradiology with the same accuracy as a neuroradiologist reporting conventional images. Teleradiology in stroke is discussed further in Chapter 6.

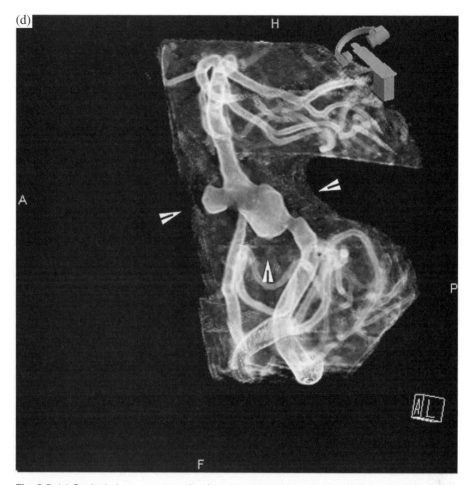

Fig. 8.5. (a) Sagittal-plane reconstruction from a computed tomography (CT) angiographic study. A bi-lobar aneurysm can be seen, involving the distal left vertebral artery and proximal basilar artery (arrows). (b) Sagittal-plane fluid-attenuated inversion-recovery (FLAIR) magnetic resonance image, showing a large partially thrombosed aneurysm sac (arrowhead) indenting the medulla oblongata. (c) Digital subtraction angiogram, left vertebral artery injection. The large posterior lobe and smaller anterior lobe of the aneurysm are visualized (arrowheads). (d) Computer-generated three-dimensional (3D) reconstruction of rotational angiographic data. The ability to rotate the data set in 3D space allows the aneurysm to be characterized fully in relation to branch vessels and endovascular accessibility.

Another way of transmitting neuroradiology images is with a document camera attached to videoconferencing equipment, which enables real-time transfer of the image to videoconferencing equipment at a distant site. Although no formal reliability studies of this method have been published, it has been used in clinical practice to administer IV tPA.[13]

Teleradiology also can be used in less urgent cases, when the opinion of a neurologist or a neuroradiologist may be sought to assist in the diagnosis or the management of a patient, as in the following case report.

Case report 2

A 16-year-old girl presented to a neurologist with short stature and delayed puberty. She was noted to be anosmic and was diagnosed as suffering from hypogonadotrophic hypogonadism. She was commenced on low-dose oestrogen as hormone replacement, but within two weeks she began to complain of headaches, nausea and memory lapses. On admission to hospital two weeks later, she had clinical signs of a right-sided cranial lesion. An MR study showed features of cerebral infarction (Fig. 8.6a,b). The cause of

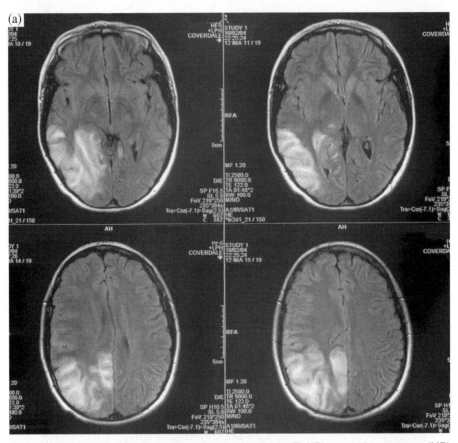

Fig. 8.6. (a) Axial-plane fluid-attenuated inversion-recovery (FLAIR) magnetic resonance (MR) image, showing bright signal intensity of recent right parieto-occipital infarction. (b) Axial-plane B1000 image, confirming the restricted diffusion of acute infarct. (c) MR angiogram, showing abnormal bright signal intensity (arrowhead) and pruning of posterior parietal branches of the middle cerebral artery (arrow).

(b)

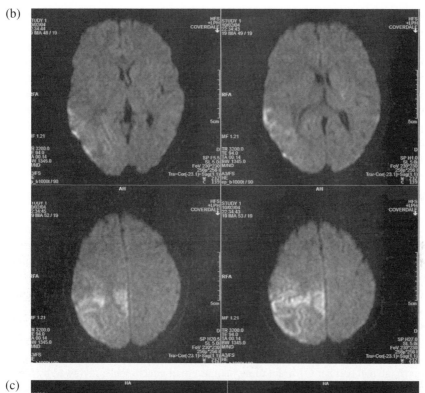

(c)

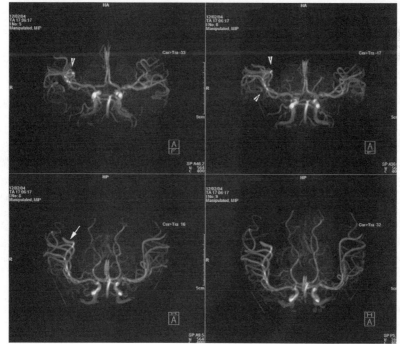

the infarct was not identified, but dural venous thrombosis infarction was considered in the context of oestrogen ingestion.

The images were transferred to a subspecialist neuroradiologist at a tertiary hospital 110 km away for review. He confirmed the dural venous sinuses to be normal but considered the MR angiogram to be abnormal (Fig. 8.6c). The possibility of mitochondrial encephalopathy was raised, prompting blood lactate measurement, which was abnormally high. Further investigation confirmed the diagnosis as mitochondrial encephalopathy with lactic acidosis and stroke-like episodes (MELAS syndrome). The patient did not require transfer for diagnosis.

Developing world

The telecommunications infrastructure necessary for teleradiology does not exist in much of the developing world, although CT and MRI scanners often do. Alternative methods of image transfer must be applied in this situation. The use of a digital camera to photograph radiological images on a light box has been described.[14,15] Corr and colleagues[14] found that pathology on 6% of the digital camera images was missed (in comparison with reading the original image). These missed pathologies were all subtle. Patterson and colleagues[15] described the digital camera pictures of MR and CT scans sent as email attachments as 'easily interpretable by the neurologist'. A case study by Graham and colleagues[16] described positive outcomes for a Nepalese patient who suffered a spontaneous cerebral haemorrhage and had her CT brain films, sent as email attachments, reviewed by a neurologist, neurosurgeon and neuroradiologist in Belfast some 8000 km away. Advice from these specialists was then sent back to the referring doctor in Nepal by email. The use of email is described in more detail in Chapters 3 and 10.

Intercontinental teleradiology

Teleradiology can also be used to take advantage of world time-zone differences. Developments in telecommunications mean that broadband Internet connections are now readily available and can be used to transfer medical images at clinically acceptable speeds. Kalyanpur and colleagues[17] described how US hospitals used an external teleradiology service provider to provide review of emergency CT scans by a US-board-certified radiologist working in Bangalore, India. The night shift (23.00–07.00) in the USA corresponds with the day shift (08.00–16.00) in Bangalore. CT scans are performed in the USA; the images are then transmitted to India for reporting, and the resultant radiologist's report is transferred back to the referring doctor in the USA. For CT head scans reported via this teleradiology service, the final radiologist's report was available in less than 40 minutes, which included an image-transmission time of six minutes. It is interesting to note that despite the great intercontinental distance, the turnaround time for reporting was less than that reported in the Austrian study.[11]

Conclusion

Teleradiology is an integral part of the practice of not only neuroradiology but also neurosurgery and neurology. The technology, whether based on a PACS or a web-server, is increasingly being incorporated into neurological healthcare systems worldwide. The use of telemedicine in neuroradiology has achieved the goal of telemedicine in general in bringing together medical experts with patients who need their services, even when they are separated by distance and possibly by time. Teleneuroradiology should serve as a model for other applications of telemedicine within clinical neuroscience.

Further information

ACR/NEMA DICOM standard. http://medical.nema.org. The standard can be downloaded in PDF format from this site. Accessed 4 February 2005.

University of Iowa Hospitals and Clinics, Department of Radiology. An introduction to teleradiology. www.radiology.uiowa.edu/MoreRAD/Teleradiology/Tele.html. This includes product comparisons of commercially available teleradiology products. Accessed 4 February 2005.

PACSpage. PACS/telemedicine resource page. www.dejarnette.com/efinegan/pacspage.htm. A table-of-contents website with links to many useful DICOM, PACS and teleradiology websites. Accessed 4 February 2005.

References

1   Jutras A. Teleroentgen diagnosis by means of video-tape recording. *American Journal of Roentgenology, Radium Therapy, and Nuclear Medicine* 1959; 82: 1099–102.
2   Erickson BJ. *Irreversible Compression of Medical Images.* Society for Computer Applications in Radiology. www.scarnet.org/pdf/scarwhitepaper.pdf. Accessed 3 February 2005.
3   American College of Radiologists. *ACR Technical Standard for Teleradiology* www.acr.org/s_acr/bin.asp?trackid=&sid=1&did=12292&cid=541&vid=2&doc=file.pdf. Accessed 3 February 2005.
4   Servadei F, Antonelli V, Mastrilli A *et al.* Integration of image transmission into a protocol for head injury management: a preliminary report. *British Journal of Neurosurgery* 2002; **16**: 36–42.
5   Jithoo R, Govender PV, Corr P, Nathoo N. Telemedicine and neurosurgery: experience of a regional unit based in South Africa. *Journal of Telemedicine and Telecare* 2003; **9**: 63–66.
6   Hazebroucq V, Fery-Lemonnier E. The value of teleradiology in the management of neuroradiologic emergencies. [Article in French] *Journal of Neuroradiology* 2004; **31**: 334–339.
7   Stormo A, Sollid S, Stormer J, Ingebrigsten T. Neurosurgical teleconsultations in northern Norway. *Journal of Telemedicine and Telecare* 2004; **10**; 135–139.
8   Poon WS, Goh KY. The impact of teleradiology on the inter-hospital transfer of neurosurgical patients and their outcome. *Hong Kong Medical Journal* 1998; **4**: 293–295.
9   Schwamm LH, Rosenthal ES, Hirshberg A *et al.* Virtual TeleStroke support for the emergency department evaluation of acute stroke. *Academic Emergency Medicine* 2004; **11**: 1193–1197.
10 Levine SR, Gorman M. 'Telestroke': the application of telemedicine for stroke. *Stroke* 1999; **30**: 464–469.
11 Soegner P, Rettenbacher T, Smekal A *et al.* Benefit for the patient of a teleradiology process certified to meet an international standard. *Journal of Telemedicine and Telecare* 2003; 9 (suppl. 2): 61–62.
12 Johnston KC, Worrall BB. Teleradiology Assessment of Computerized Tomographs Online Reliability Study (TRACTORS) for acute stroke evaluation. *Telemedicine Journal and e-Health* 2003; **9**: 227–233.

13   Choi JY, Wojner AW, Cale RT *et al.* Telemedicine physician providers: augmented acute stroke care delivery in rural Texas: an initial experience. *Telemedicine Journal and e-Health* 2004; **10** (suppl. 2): 90–94.

14   Corr P, Couper I, Beningfield SJ, Mars M. A simple telemedicine system using a digital camera. *Journal of Telemedicine and Telecare* 2000; **6**: 233–236.

15   Patterson V, Hoque F, Vassallo D *et al.* Store-and-forward teleneurology in developing countries. *Journal of Telemedicine and Telecare* 2001; **7** (suppl. 1): 52–53.

16   Graham LE, Flynn P, Cooke S, Patterson V. The interdisciplinary management of cerebral haemorrhage using telemedicine: a case report from Nepal. *Journal of Telemedicine and Telecare* 2001: **7**: 304–306.

17   Kalyanpur A, Weinberg J, Neklesa V *et al.* Emergency radiology coverage: technical and clinical feasibility of an international teleradiology model. *Emergency Radiology* 2003; **10**: 115–118.

▶9

Telemedicine and Clinical Neurophysiology

Sean Connolly and Mary Fitzsimons

Background

In clinical neurophysiology (CN), electrodiagnostic procedures are used to evaluate the integrity and function of the nervous system, including the brain, spinal cord, peripheral nerves and muscles. There is a shortage of CN specialists in most parts of the world, so it is not possible to provide CN services everywhere. Telemedicine can be used to improve access to shared and remote CN expertise. Teleneurophysiology services can speed up diagnosis and result in more patients being investigated appropriately. It may also provide a more accessible CN service by decentralizing specialist care.

Clinical neurophysiology

The routine investigations carried out in a CN department include electroencephalography (EEG), nerve conduction studies (NCS), needle electromyography (EMG) and evoked potential (EP) recordings. These tests, carried out on inpatients and outpatients, are used to record and display bioelectric signals originating in the brain, along nerve pathways and in muscles. The acquired signals, transduced by electrodes, are amplified and displayed visually for interpretation. Current CN technology allows the signals to be recorded and stored on a digital medium, such as a hard disk, compact disk (CD) or digital versatile disk (DVD).

These routine investigations can take 30–120 minutes to perform. Some additional, more advanced CN investigations, such as quantitative EMG, long-term monitoring for epilepsy, intraoperative monitoring and intensive care unit (ICU) monitoring, are more time-consuming and require additional specific expertise from technicians and CN consultants. Most CN investigations are compatible with teleneurophysiology.

The Association of British Clinical Neurophysiologists (ABCN) estimates that a service with a capacity to perform 1600 CN tests per annum is required per 250 000 population.[1] This would comprise 800 EEGs, 600 NCSs/EMGs and 200 EPs.

Investigations

The four main investigations in CN are:

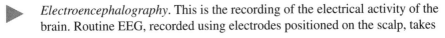 *Electroencephalography.* This is the recording of the electrical activity of the brain. Routine EEG, recorded using electrodes positioned on the scalp, takes

approximately one hour to complete. The main indications for EEG referral are to investigate epilepsy and disorders of consciousness. It is also used in the diagnosis and management of encephalopathies and neurodegenerative disorders. Modern EEG recording incorporates synchronous video recording of the patient in order to correlate electrographic activity with any clinical change.

▶ *Nerve conduction studies (NCSs).* These involve electrically stimulating a nerve at one location and recording either the resultant nerve action potential (NAP) as it passes another location (in the case of a sensory nerve) or the evoked compound muscle action potential (CMAP) from a muscle innervated by a motor nerve (Fig. 9.1). The stimulation and recording can be made by means of electrodes that are placed on the skin surface overlying the nerve or muscle. NCSs can be used to determine the site and nature of pathological processes affecting peripheral nerve conduction.

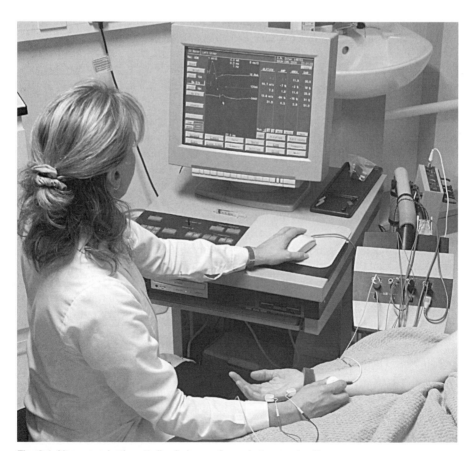

Fig. 9.1. Nerve conduction studies being performed at a remote site.

▶ *Electromyography.* This is the recording of spontaneous and voluntary electrical activity produced by skeletal muscles. EMG is usually recorded by means of a needle electrode inserted into the muscle of interest. It is used to identify and characterize diseases of the muscles, neuromuscular junctions and peripheral nerves.

▶ *Evoked potential studies.* These are used to measure the integrity of sensory and motor pathways of the nervous system. The conduction of signals along sensory nerve pathways to the brain can be measured by placing electrodes on the skin over the relevant neural routes. The potentials are used to differentiate between abnormalities in the peripheral and central portions of the nerve pathways. They are of particular benefit in providing an objective means of measuring sensory pathway function. Frequently used EPs include visual evoked responses (VERs), brainstem auditory evoked responses (BAERs) and somatosensory evoked potentials (SSEPs). Motor EPs recorded from limb muscles can be elicited non-invasively by electrical or magnetic stimulation of the motor cortex and spinal roots.

Clinical neurophysiology service

The majority of CN investigations are carried out in an outpatient setting. Patients are referred for investigation from hospital consultants, mainly neurologists, paediatricians, general physicians, psychiatrists, rheumatologists, neurosurgeons and orthopaedic surgeons. Referrals also may come from primary-care doctors.

A CN service is usually provided by a suitably qualified medical consultant and supported by neurophysiological measurement technicians. EEG and EP recordings can be made by trained technicians but normally are interpreted by CN consultants. Needle EMG recordings can be conducted only by CN consultants. Often, NCS and EMG recordings form parts of a single investigation conducted by the CN consultant. Many NCSs can be conducted by trained technicians under consultant supervision. In this way, an NCS clinic can investigate patients referred for investigation of certain disorders, such as carpal tunnel syndrome and peripheral neuropathy. It is crucial that the technicians receive appropriate direction and supervision from a CN consultant to ensure a high-quality service.

Teleneurophysiology

In practical terms, teleneurophysiology involves a technician at a remote department recording CN data (Fig. 9.1). The recorded digital data are then accessed by a specialist centre for interpretation by a CN consultant and a report is sent back to the remote department. Data transfer can be accomplished either via a telecommunication link or by conveying a digital storage medium to the specialist centre.

Service organization

Teleneurophysiology will require a main department to be connected to a number of remote or satellite departments. Recordings that do not require the on-site presence of a CN consultant can be made by well-trained technicians at the satellite departments and interpreted by the clinician at the main department. This can apply to routine EEGs, most EPs and many NCSs.

Remote access can be provided to previously stored digital data and to data during acquisition. Thus, the CN consultant at the main department can log on to a server to review previously recorded data and to monitor acquisitions that are currently in progress. As a result, unnecessary duplication of data can be avoided, and investigations can be reviewed easily and quickly. Clinical reports can be sent electronically to the relevant satellite site. Such a CN network can be local, regional, national or international.

Transmission considerations

The telecommunications infrastructure required for teleneurophysiology is determined by the size of the CN data files, the acquisition rate of the digital data and the requirements for dynamic data review. These factors will dictate the bandwidth of the required network and, hence, the cost.

Digital CN data-file sizes depend on the number of channels required, the sampling rate and resolution of the analogue-to-digital conversion of the bioelectric signal, and the duration of the recording. File sizes from tens of kilobytes for simple NCS and EP studies up to the order of 50 MB for one hour of continuous EEG recording are common. A digital video recording accompanying the EEG will produce a file of approximately 1 GB.

Telecommunication options include the ordinary public switched telephone networks (PSTNs) transmitting at a maximum of 56 kbit/s, the digital equivalent (integrated services digital network, ISDN) transmitting at rates from 64 kbit/s to 2 Mbit/s, and asynchronous digital subscriber lines (ADSL) transmitting at rates of 512 kbit/s or higher.

Tele-electroencephalography

Because of the very large file sizes, implementing tele-EEG in practice is not easy. Although there were reports of the feasibility of EEG transmission over the telephone network as early as 1969,[2] there is remarkably little literature on tele-EEG, either experimentally or in clinical practice. Digital photography can be used to send single EEG pages as email attachments, and this was employed successfully between a mobile telemedicine unit in north-west Russia and Tromsø in Norway.[3] Data-compression algorithms are available that allow transmission of EEGs over a public telephone network with a transmission time of 2.2 seconds per page. The compression used to enable this did not seem to affect interpretation of the EEG.[4] The authors commented that review of EEG at one page every two seconds was vastly preferable to having to drive to work to review an urgent record. Transmission of full EEG files, with or without video, requires a network operating at 10–100 Mbit/s. Loula and colleagues[5] reported on a consultation forum in Finland based on a high-speed fibre-optic network that resulted in numerous benefits for participating hospitals.

Tele-EEG is worthwhile for a number of reasons: EEGs can be carried out closer to the homes of many patients, neonatal EEGs can be interpreted by appropriately trained experts, urgent cases (such as status epilepticus) can be interpreted promptly, perioperative electrocorticography can be assessed from an office, continuing medical education (CME) for technicians working alone in remote departments is enhanced, and multicentre review of EEG records is possible.

Web-based systems

One method of implementing remote access teleneurophysiology is to use a web-based CN service. This has the advantage that it would be scalable, allowing multiple CN sites to be connected to a network (Fig. 9.2). Digital data acquired at the satellite CN departments would be sent via a secure network to a central server.

Access to a web-based network could be via the public Internet or, as in the Swedish example described below, by means of a separate intranet. If the public Internet is employed, then secure communication can be ensured by use of a virtual private network (VPN), which provides an encrypted data 'tunnel' through the public Internet. CN consultants with the appropriate expertise – eg adult or paediatric EEG or EMG – can access the data via a workstation for interpretation. The bandwidth of the network

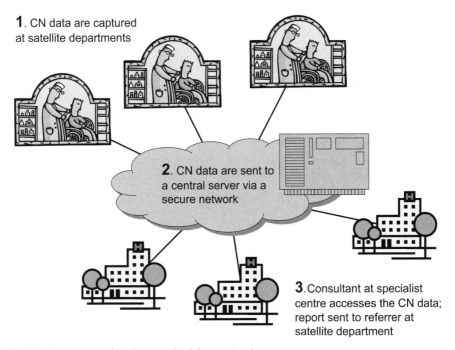

1. CN data are captured at satellite departments

2. CN data are sent to a central server via a secure network

3. Consultant at specialist centre accesses the CN data; report sent to referrer at satellite department

Fig. 9.2. Architecture of a teleneurophysiology network.
CN, clinical neurophysiology

and the performance of the reporting workstation must meet data review and display standards.[4] Having interpreted the data, a report can be sent electronically to referring physicians and the satellite CN department. Web-based operations are not limited by the location of the satellite department or the reporting consultant.

Compatibility

Interoperability of the CN systems in a teleneurophysiology service is important, since centres may have CN equipment from a variety of manufacturers. The development of standards for digital CN data will facilitate the exchange of bioelectric signals between the centres. This is essential so that the review software is capable of reliably displaying the neurophysiological data acquired at the satellite sites.

Videoconferencing

A teleneurophysiology service can be enhanced by videoconferencing facilities in the CN departments in combination with biosignal transmission. Videoconferencing allows geographically separated clinicians and technicians to participate in joint reporting sessions, case conferences, training sessions, lectures and departmental conferences, which will result in improved CN standards; see Chapter 4 for further details.

Example of teleneurophysiology

A well-developed example of teleneurophysiology exists between Uppsala University Hospital in Sweden and other regional hospitals throughout Sweden and the Baltic states[6–8]. Satellite CN services in the regions are linked to the specialist centre at Uppsala via an intranet, known as Sjunet, which is separate from the Internet. Sjunet is the Swedish healthcare network. The precursor to Sjunet was the Baltic International Telemedicine Network (BITNET), which incorporated multiple medical applications, including a teleneurophysiology collaboration between Uppsala University Hospital and Estonia, Latvia and Lithuania. The pioneering work of BITNET prompted the establishment of Sjunet, a broadband network that provides infrastructure for secure transmission of data and applications between hospitals, primary-care centres and home care. The network facilitates a number of telemedicine activities, including videoconferencing, teleradiology, database access and secure email messaging, as well as teleneurophysiology.

In the Uppsala-based teleneurophysiology service, CN data (eg EEG, NCS) are acquired by technicians at the satellite centres. Analysis of the data is performed by a CN consultant at the university hospital. Acquired digital data are stored on a local server at the satellite centre and the CN consultant accesses the local server through the network to review the data. After analysis of the data, a report is generated, which is sent to the referring physician by email. This procedure means that clinical data recorded at the satellite centres are archived in databases at that location. A videoconferencing facility links the specialist centre with the satellite centres. This provides additional benefits in terms of education and sharing of knowledge and in improving CN standards.

Benefits of teleneurophysiology

The introduction of teleneurophysiology services will allow patients to have local access to certain CN services, referring clinicians to have increased support from colleagues in expert centres, and healthcare managers to improve integration of services and so reduce waiting lists and associated costs. There will be more efficient use of specialists' time because of reduced travel between sites. Quality of service should improve with immediate consultations for remote colleagues and the possibility of on-call EEG services with national or international collaboration. All of this should lead to more cost-effective practice.

Consideration of teleneurophysiology is timely, since many countries are trying to exploit information and communication technology (ICT) to improve information management and to support advances in healthcare delivery, eg electronic health records and telemedicine.[9] Advances in ICT are likely to revolutionize healthcare and make health services more accessible and responsive by bringing expertise closer to people, especially those in remote locations.

Teleneurophysiology service evaluation

A teleneurophysiology service will not be located in a single hospital but will connect healthcare providers to patients and healthcare professionals at many different locations. It thus breaks down traditional organizational boundaries. Such a service has the potential to improve quality and value for money through better use of healthcare resources. However, careful consideration must be given to the changes required to the traditional delivery and management structures. It is also important to evaluate teleneurophysiology services. This means establishing a pre-implementation baseline against which post-implementation changes can be appraised. Without evaluation aimed at understanding the criteria for success, healthcare policy-makers and managers should be cautious about recommending increased use and investment in ICT.[10] Healthcare developments must be driven by the needs of the service users rather than the technology.

Assessment of needs

In preparation for the introduction of a teleneurophysiology service in Ireland, we conducted a study of the need for CN services and the feasibility of teleneurophysiology to provide them.[11,12] The study was conducted in two parts. First, we compared CN referral profiles of patients in a large urban region with local services with those of patients in a rural region without services. Second, we examined patients' and referring physicians' needs, expectations and satisfaction with existing CN services. For residents of the CN-deficient region, there was a distance of more than 240 km to the nearest service.

Patients in rural regions were likely to wait longer for an appointment compared with their urban equivalents. Physicians in the rural area, although they considered CN investigations important in patient management, felt discouraged from referring their patients, because of the long distances involved and because delays caused by long waiting lists made referral irrelevant (Table 9.1). In addition, the ratio of adult to

Table 9.1. Responses (*n*, % of total) to referring clinician satisfaction survey

	Yes	No	Occasionally		Total no. of respondents
Is CN relevant to your medical practice?	27 (90)	1 (3)	2 (7)		30
	EEG	**EMG/NCS**	**EP**	**All**	
Which CN investigation are you most likely to use?	12 (40)	8 (27)	1 (3)	9 (30)	30
	Dublin	**Galway**	**Dublin/Galway**		
Where are your patients referred to for CN investigation?	16 (67)	1 (4)	7 (29)		24
	< 1 month	**1–3 months**	**> 3 months**		
What is the average waiting time for CN testing experienced by your patients?	4 (17)	9 (39)	10 (44)		23
	< 25%	**25–49%**	**50–75%**	**> 75%**	
What proportion of CN tests are considered helpful in patient management?	2 (8)	9 (38)	5 (21)	8 (33)	24
	Yes	**No**	**Sometimes**		
Are CN reports readily available at follow-up appointments with patients?	11 (44)	12 (48)	2 (8)		25
	Yes	**No**			
Are you happy with the availability of CN services?	1 (3)	28 (97)			29
	Yes	**No**			
Does lack of a local service affect patient management negatively?	30 (97)	1 (3)			31
	Always	**Sometimes**	**Never**		
Does lack of a local service dissuade referral?	10 (33)	14 (47)	6 (20)		30
	Yes	**No**			
Would you welcome the introduction of a teleneurophysiology service?	27 (93)	2 (7)			29
	Yes	**No**			
Are there any negative implications about the introduction of teleneurophysiology?	12 (46)	14 (54)			26

CN, clinical neurophysiology; EEG, electroencephalography; EMG, electromyography; EP, evoked potential; NCS, nerve conduction studies.

paediatric patients referred for CN suggested an underuse of services for adults living in the rural region. Older people were particularly reluctant to travel for testing.

The referring physicians from the rural region felt that the lack of local access to services impeded patient management (Table 9.1). They welcomed the introduction of a teleneurophysiology service, as it would result in more patients being investigated appropriately. Where negative concerns about introducing teleneurophysiology were expressed, these related to the assurance of the calibre of technical personnel delivering the satellite service and the need for paediatric EEGs to be interpreted by appropriately experienced CN consultants. Achieving and maintaining high levels of professional competence were recognized as challenges to be met in delivering telemedicine services.[13]

Other issues

Teleneurophysiology has the potential to address service inequities. However, in implementing a teleneurophysiology service, the legal and ethical issues, security, and standards for the management of digital data in health must be considered. It is essential that at least the same quality of care, duty of care and interprofessional relationships is delivered as with conventional healthcare delivery. Adherence to relevant data-protection legislation is essential to uphold individuals' privacy and confidentiality. Because traditional institutional boundaries are crossed in telemedicine services, legal responsibility for the service may require additional attention. Finally, electronic data are vulnerable to attacks, including from unauthorized personnel and computer viruses.

Conclusion

For over 40 years, progress in CN has paralleled technological advance. This has been particularly apparent in the past decade, and most CN departments are now based on digital equipment. In the past 15 years, the rapid development of the Internet has seen its application in healthcare advance from email to the advent of departmental websites that provide information for patients, referring clinicians and other departments world-wide. Clinicians in remote sites can be supported by email, videoconferencing and websites. The increasing availability of broadband and other telecommunications infrastructure in many countries should facilitate this progress. Integrating these technical advances to produce a teleneurophysiology service is certainly possible. Its feasibility and potential benefits are evinced by the Swedish and Baltic experiences.

Further information

Hailey D, Roine R, Ohinmaa A. Systematic review of evidence for the benefits of telemedicine. *Journal of Telemedicine and Telecare* 2002; **8** (suppl. 1): 1–30.

Stålberg E, Stålberg S. Regional network in clinical neurophysiology, tele-EMG. In *European Telemedicine 1998/99*. Wootton R, ed. London: Kensington Publications, 1999; pp. 101–103.

Project on Telemedicine: Regional and National Collaboration. *What are the Barriers Facing Telemedicine?* www.carelink.se/files/doc_200364153958.pdf. Accessed 3 February 2005.

Stanberry B. *Legal and Ethical Aspects of Telemedicine.* London: Royal Society of Medicine Press, 1998.

References

1   Association of British Clinical Neurophysiologists. *Clinical Neurophysiology Specialty Statement.* London: Association of British Clinical Neurophysiologists, 2001.
2   Hanley J, Zweizig JR, Kado RT *et al.* Combined telephone and radiotelemetry of the EEG. *Electroencephalography and Clinical Neurophysiology* 1969; **26**: 323–324.
3   Uldal SB, Amerkhanov J, Manankova Bye S *et al.* A mobile telemedicine unit for emergency and screening purposes: experience from north-west Russia. *Journal of Telemedicine and Telecare* 2004; **10**: 11–15.
4   Holder D, Cameron J, Binnie C. Tele-EEG in epilepsy: review and initial experience with software to enable EEG review over a telephone link. *Seizure* 2003; **12**: 85–91.
5   Loula P, Rauhala E, Erkinjuntti M *et al.* Distributed clinical neurophysiology. *Journal of Telemedicine and Telecare* 1997; **3**: 89–95.
6   Stålberg E. The integrated digital clinical neurophysiology laboratory. In *Clinical Neurophysiology, Vol. 2: EEG, Paediatric Neurophysiology, Special Techniques and Applications.* Binnie C, Cooper R, Maugière *et al.*, eds. London: Elsevier, 2003; pp. 971–98.
7   Stålberg S. Small bits to big bites. *Muscle and Nerve* 2002; **25** (suppl. 11): 119–127.
8   Jabre JF, Stålberg EV, Bassi R. Telemedicine and internet EMG. In *Clinical Neurophysiology at the Beginning of the 21st Century.* Ambler Z, Nevšímalová S, Kadaňka Z, Rossine PM, eds. Amsterdam: Elsevier Science, 2000; pp. 163–167.
9   McConnell H. International efforts in implementing national health information infrastructure and electronic health records. *World Hospitals and Health Services* 2004; **40**: 33–7, 39–40, 50–52.
10   Currell R, Urquhart C, Wainwright P, Lewis R. Telemedicine versus face to face patient care: effects on professional practice and health care outcomes. *Cochrane Database of Systematic Reviews* 2000; **2**: CD002098.
11   Fitzsimons M, Ronan L, Murphy K *et al.* Customer needs, expectations, and satisfaction with clinical neurophysiology services in Ireland: a case for tele-neurophysiology development. *Irish Medical Journal* 2004; **97**: 208–211.
12   Ronan L, Murphy K, Browne G *et al.* Needs analysis for tele-neurophysiology in the Irish North-Western Health Board. *Irish Medical Journal* 2004; **97**: 46–49.
13   Roberts GH, Dunscombe PB, Samant RS. Geographic delivery models for radiotherapy services. *Australasian Radiology* 2002; **46**: 290–294.

▶10

Teleneurology in the Developing World

Victor Patterson, Mostafa Kamal and Stephen Read

Introduction

Neurological diseases are common worldwide. However, they are more prevalent in the developing world, mainly because of the increased occurrence there of infectious diseases, such as polio, leprosy, human immunodeficiency virus (HIV)/acquired immunodeficiency syndrome (AIDS) and malaria.[1,2] In addition, the developing world has all the neurological diseases of the industrialized world – brain tumours and strokes, epilepsy and tension headaches, hysterical disorders and Parkinson's disease.

There are far fewer doctors in the developing world than in the industrialized world, and most tend to live in big cities, which has the effect of leaving rural communities underserved. The number of neurologists is even fewer, and many countries do not have any neurologists at all.[3] Since neurologists almost certainly improve the outcomes of people with neurological diseases, finding a way to bring more neurological expertise to bear on patients with neurological disorders in the developing world is a problem worth solving.

One obvious solution is to train more doctors in general, and more neurologists in particular, and then somehow induce them to live in rural areas. However, this could only bear fruit in the long term and may also be somewhat unrealistic in practice. The question is whether telemedicine can help in the short to medium term.

Telemedicine as a solution

Technical considerations

There are two types of telemedicine: real-time telemedicine delivered either by telephone or videoconferencing, and asynchronous telemedicine delivered by email or the Internet. Both types require an underlying communications infrastructure, which represents a problem in developing countries, where access to telephones is often poor. Integrated services digital network (ISDN) lines and broadband connections are beginning to be introduced, but they are still extremely expensive. The reliability of connections to other countries is often poor. In contrast, almost all countries have access to an Internet service provider, and these have become more reliable in recent years, so that their service is less likely to be crashed by large email attachments.

Real-time teleneurology by telephone

Telephone neurology is one possible solution. Use of the telephone for telemedicine is attractive, as international call charges continue to decline in price. The telephone also has the advantage that there can be interaction between the doctors involved. On the debit side, a full neurological consultation will take perhaps 20–30 minutes, especially between doctors who do not know each other and are talking about a complicated patient; it may also be difficult to find a mutually convenient time for two doctors in different time zones to communicate. Besides, real-time teleneurology by telephone between doctors has not caught on in the industrialized world, so it is difficult to see why it should be any more popular in the developing world (see Chapter 2).

Real-time teleneurology by videolink

Real-time teleneurology would normally be between a specialist in the industrialized world and the referring doctor together with the patient in the developing world. This is the most comprehensive telemedicine option and enables the neurologist to take the history (if necessary, through an interpreter) and witness the examination. Again, however, scheduling a suitable time may be difficult, the consultation is likely to take more than 30 minutes, and even if the necessary ISDN lines are available it will be expensive. Also, because of the poor availability of ISDN services, it is likely to be applicable only to hospitals in large centres.

In principle the Internet can be used for real-time teleneurology, but in practice there seems to be no experience of this. It is unlikely that good-quality video pictures could be transmitted reliably across the Internet in its present form.

Asynchronous teleneurology by Web access

In asynchronous telemedicine using the Web, the referring doctor connects to the Internet and fills in a Web-based proforma, which is then dealt with by a specialist or a series of specialists in the industrialized world. This is not likely to be generally applicable for teleneurology, since Web access is not readily available everywhere and is also considerably more expensive in terms of telephone costs than ordinary email.

Asynchronous teleneurology by email

The lowest-cost option is to use the telephone network for sending email. Most information about a patient can be written down, so email is an excellent medium for this purpose. Images of patients or their radiological investigations can be attached to email messages. Email allows the replying doctor to choose a place and time of reply. It usually takes 10–20 minutes to send a reply, depending on the complexity of the problem. Even though the mode of communication is asynchronous, it is still possible for the referring doctor to receive a reply by the next day, or even quicker. Email is more reliable than it used to be, doctors are familiar with it in other parts of their lives, and it is relatively inexpensive (in terms of call charges) to send and receive messages.

Use of telemedicine in the developing world

All specialties

There are surprisingly few studies of telemedicine in the developing world, and all have used asynchronous communication. The Swinfen Charitable Trust (SCT), a UK-based medical charity, has established email links between a number of hospitals in the developing world and a network of specialists in the industrialized world (Box 10.1). It has reported its initial experience in Bangladesh[4] and its later experience in Nepal.[5] In the Bangladesh experience, 24 of 27 referrals were felt by the referring doctor to have benefited, with four being spared the expense of having to travel abroad. In Nepal, an independent assessment judged that the email telemedicine service shortened hospital stay in 50% of patients. A Web-based system has been used in Vietnam[6] and also in Cambodia, where there is a tripartite service between a rural village (Robib), a hospital in Phnom Penh and the Massachusetts General Hospital in Boston, USA.[7]

Box 10.1 The Swinfen Charitable Trust (SCT)

The SCT is a registered UK charity whose aims are 'assisting poor, sick and disabled people in the developing world'. One method by which it does this is telemedicine, which is used to provide online advice to hospital doctors in developing countries.

The SCT supplies referring doctors with a computer, digital camera and accessories, and trains the local staff in their use. The hospital provides access to a dial-up Internet service provider for the transmission and receipt of email. Web access is not used, because it is not affordable in the hospitals of most developing countries.

The SCT is an apolitical, non-religious organization. It receives funding through donations from the general public. Its staff members are unpaid volunteers. The online consultations are supplied by a global network of consultant-grade specialists, most of whom live in industrialized countries.

The SCT receives many requests from hospitals in developing countries to join the network. A condition of entry is that poor patients are treated free of charge. At present, the SCT helps 43 hospitals in 18 countries.

See www.uq.edu.au/swinfen for further details.

Teleneurology

Only the SCT has reported any separate experience within neurology.[8] Twelve patients who were managed by email were judged by the neurologist as extremely complex. He felt secure in his diagnosis in only four cases and would have felt much happier with a real-time videolink in the others. However, the doctor in the developing world felt that the advice received was helpful in 11 of 12 cases. This perceptual difference was crucially important in encouraging the continued practice of email teleneurology to the developing world. The rest of this chapter is devoted to reporting the results.

Process of email teleneurology

Referring hospitals are equipped by the SCT with a portable computer, a digital camera and a tripod. The local staff members are trained in the use of this equipment and how to use it so that patient anonymity is protected (Fig. 10.1).[4] To make a referral, the referring doctor summarizes the case and asks the specialist the relevant questions. Any clinical or X-ray images are attached to the email message, which is then sent to a single email address, the SCT AutoRouter, which is a message-handling computer managed by people and located in Brisbane, Australia (Fig. 10.2).[9] The system administrators, who are located in different time zones, check the server for referrals periodically throughout the 24-hour day and direct them to appropriate specialists. This system was introduced in 2002 because the manual system was becoming difficult to operate due to the increased number of referrals. The AutoRouter is programmed to identify any replies not made within 48 hours and either to send a follow-up email message or to redirect the original referral to another specialist. It

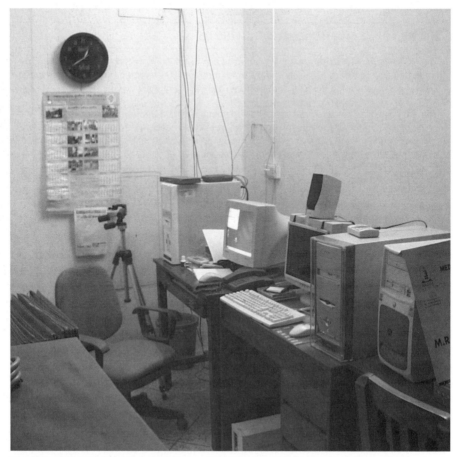

Fig. 10.1. Telemedicine office at Centre for Rehabilitation of the Paralysed, Bangladesh.

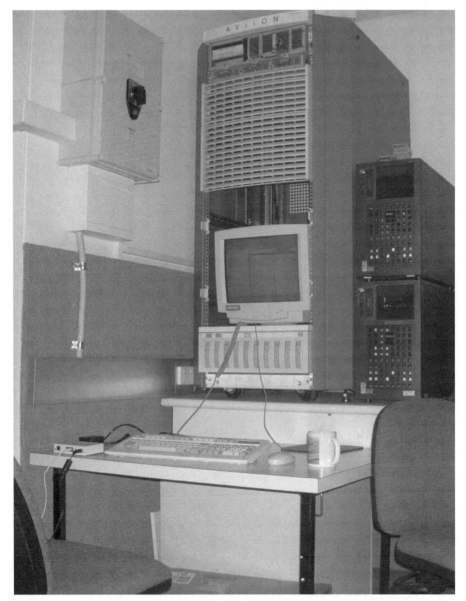

Fig. 10.2. Swinfen Charitable Trust AutoRouter (automatic message-handling system).

makes the data both secure and accessible and provides a solution to an important administrative problem.

The neurologist receives the email at an address, or addresses, which he or she has chosen. Once the neurologist makes their response, they simply forward this to the AutoRouter by clicking on the Reply icon in their email software. The message is received by the AutoRouter and routed automatically to the originator of the request. This system is shown diagrammatically in Fig. 10.3 and the functions of each component are shown in Table 10.1.

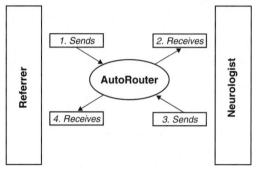

Fig. 10.3. Summary of referral process.

Table 10.1. Teleneurology process

Referring hospital:
- identifies patient
- summarizes details in email
- takes digital photos of X-rays or patient
- sends email

AutoRouter:
- receives email
- allocates a number
- refers to appropriate consultant
- identifies if no reply and redirects

Neurologist:
- receives email
- replies to AutoRouter

Email teleneurology results

Neurology represents the second most frequently requested opinion after orthopaedics, with 100 referrals having been made up to January 2005. Complete data exist on 76 adult patients. We have carried out three studies on these patients. First, we performed a retrospective analysis of the neurological cases with complete data. Second, we compared a small group of patients who were examined both face-to-face and using email. Third, we invited the referring doctors' views on the benefits of the consultations.

Retrospective review

Patients were referred from 13 hospitals from six countries, as shown in Fig. 10.4. The most frequently referring hospital was the Centre for the Rehabilitation of the

Paralysed in Dhaka, Bangladesh; the second most frequently referring hospital was the Patan Hospital in Kathmandu, Nepal. The male:female ratio of the patients was 1.8:1. The age range is shown in Fig. 10.5. The median age was 37 years.

The principal symptom for each patient was recorded (see Fig. 10.6). We also recorded secondary symptoms. When these were added to the primary group, there was a total of 15 symptoms, of which weakness was the commonest, occurring in 55% of patients.

The 15 symptoms resulted in 58 different diagnoses. These were classified into types (see Table 10.2). Disease of the lower motor unit perhaps surprisingly was the

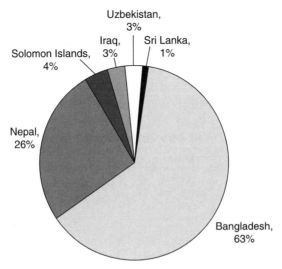

Fig. 10.4. Sources of referral (*n* = 76).

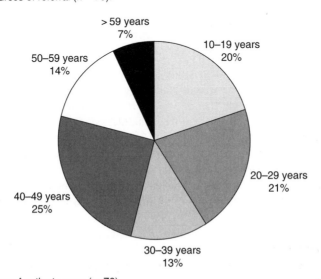

Fig. 10.5. Ages of patients seen (*n*=76).

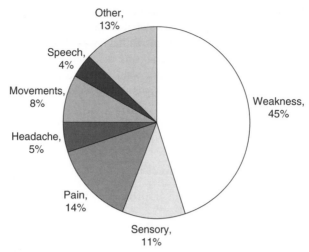

Fig. 10.6. Symptoms of patients seen (*n*=76).

Table 10.2. Types of diagnosis

Diagnosis type	*n*
Lower motor unit	25
Spinal cord	9
Cerebral	8
Degenerative	8
Stroke	6
Uncertain	6
Non-structural	3
Epilepsy	1
Other	10
Total	76

most common diagnosis, and generalized neuropathies were the most common contributor to this. Four of these neuropathies were dysimmune, and two patients had excellent responses to steroid therapy, regaining normal walking after having been confined to wheelchairs. One of these cases is described in more detail in a paper by Vassallo and colleagues.[4]

We also measured the diagnostic certainty of the neurologist on a scale between 1 (not certain at all) and 5 (very certain). The median was 4; the full results are shown in Fig. 10.7. Finally, we judged whether a video clip of the patient's gait taken on a digital camera might have helped diagnosis; this was answered positively in 23 cases. In one case, a video clip was sent.

We also assessed whether the referral had reached a natural conclusion. This was the case in 60 of the 76 patients. In the remaining 16 patients, either the neurologist did not reply to the questions or there was an indication that the patient had been discharged or died.

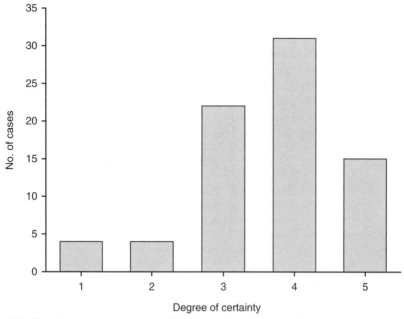

Fig. 10.7. Certainty of neurologist regarding diagnosis, on a scale from 1 (very uncertain) to 5 (very certain).

Attached clinical and radiological images were sent in 14 and 51 cases, respectively, including 32 with magnetic resonance imaging (MRI) scans; referral to a neuroradiologist was made in 16 of these patients. The method of transferring radiological data is not perfect. A single slide of each MRI sequence was sent in the first instance, with the neurologist or neuroradiologist being free to ask for subsequent digital photographs of individual slices if required.

Face-to-face validation of email diagnosis

One of us (VP) visited the Centre for the Rehabilitation of the Paralysed in Bangladesh and saw, face-to-face, five patients who had previously had an email opinion. In four patients there was complete concordance between the diagnosis by face-to-face examination and email, but in one case there was a very significant disparity (see Table 10.3). This was a seven-year-old girl in whom the email diagnosis was thought to be a

Table 10.3. Results of comparison of face-to-face diagnosis

Case	Age (years)	Sex	Email diagnosis	Face-to-face diagnosis
1	48	F	Inflammatory neuropathy	Inflammatory neuropathy
2	7	F	Quadriparesis unknown cause	Chorea
3	22	M	Spinocerebellar ataxia	Spinocerebellar ataxia
4	23	M	Cerebral degenerative disease	Cerebral degenerative disease
5	60	F	Incomplete conus lesion	Incomplete conus lesion

progressive spastic quadriparesis but who clearly had generalized chorea when seen face-to-face.

Analysis of referring doctor's views

Fifty-two patients from the Centre for the Rehabilitation of the Paralysed were assessed by the resident doctor (MK), who retrospectively reviewed the notes and recorded whether there was functional benefit, symptomatic benefit, clarification of diagnosis, clarification of management or cost-savings (see Table 10.4). Seventy-five percent of patients gained some sort of benefit, and in more than one-quarter there was a functional improvement. It is not certain, however, that this was due to the telemedicine consultation. A more narrative comment is shown in Box 10.2.

Table 10.4. Referring doctor's view of benefit ($n = 52$)

Benefit	n
Functional benefit	14
Symptomatic benefit	18
Diagnosis clarified	36
Management clarified	35
Cost-savings	19
No benefit at all	13

Box 10.2 Views of referring doctor

In Bangladesh, most people think that telemedicine is a kind of treatment and that they will be alright after receiving this treatment. In some situations, patients or their guardians show negative attitudes towards us and telemedicine when we fail to give maximum benefit in the case of non-curable disease, eg motor neurone disease. I believe that telemedicine is not magic but that we can give a lot of support to our clients with minimum cost. I think this a very good way of sharing recent ideas and treatment protocol. Through telemedicine, I have learned many things that were new to me. I think that if we can continue this programme, then we will be able to give maximum benefit to our patients.

Neurological aspects of developing-world teleneurology

The SCT referrals were exceptionally complicated neurological cases by any standard. Only three of the 76 patients had non-structural disease, which is a much lower proportion than in previously studied cohorts of inpatients,[10] outpatients[11] and referrals to accident and emergency departments.[12] Weakness usually indicates significant structural disease and was, by far, the most common symptom. In a study of email teleneurology in general practice, weakness is a symptom that has always required face-to-face examination.[13] Lower motor unit weakness was a particularly common cause; interestingly, six conditions were dysimmune and, therefore, potentially treatable. In five of these, this possibility had not been recognized before referral. In 30 of the 76 cases, the neurologist was not certain that the diagnosis was secure; an alternative way of looking at this is that the neurologist was reasonably certain of the diagnosis, and therefore the management, in 61% of patients. Epilepsy is a condition that neurologists can make a significant difference to, and the fact that only one patient with this disorder was referred indicates that we are only scratching the surface of how the industrialized world can help the developing world with neurological problems.

Telemedicine aspects

It is clear that email teleneurology is feasible. The SCT experience shows that it is possible for a rapid reply to be received, usually within one day; in 60 out of the 76 patients studied, completion was achieved. Acceptability is high in the group of referrers, but less so in the group of specialists, who are concerned about the difficulty of making accurate and therefore helpful diagnoses in many patients. A formal acceptability study has yet to be done.

That this service can be effective is indicated by the two patients in whom there was a very marked clinical improvement. Both of these patients suffered from chronic inflammatory neuropathies and made fairly impressive improvements. Also, 75% of all of the patients were judged as showing some benefit, and this is another indication of its effectiveness.

Safety information is very hard to come by in these patients, because many live a long way from the referring hospital and are lost to any sort of follow-up. Therefore, it is extremely difficult to judge the diagnostic accuracy of email teleneurology in this situation. Our cohort studied face-to-face showed good consistency in four of the five patients but a definite wrong diagnosis in one patient. Unfortunately, this sample is not large enough to make any judgement, but it is clear that in some patients the diagnosis is likely to be wrong.

A cost-effectiveness study is difficult because what is the alternative? Certainly if a patient's transfer out of the country is prevented by this service, then there is undoubtedly a saving to the patient. Our study from Nepal showed that there were reduced bed days, which indicates savings for the health provider. The great feature of email teleneurology is that the direct costs to the referrer are exceptionally small. The neurologist's time is contributed freely.

Regarding sustainability, there have been continued referrals from all the hospital sites that took part initially. In some hospitals, the referral rate has declined, which may simply be an indication that the local doctors are becoming more skilled at neurological diagnosis and management. However, the reasons for this have not been studied in sufficient detail to confirm this.

The future

It is clear that many, but not all, of these extremely complicated neurological patients can be dealt with by email teleneurology. Is this good enough? From the point of view of the developing world, it almost certainly is, because teleneurology is a service that replaces nothing and therefore any benefit must be a bonus.

Can the service be improved? There are two ways in which it might be. The first is to investigate the transmission of video clips as email attachments. This is likely to be particularly useful for patients with gait disturbance and weakness, as it should enable the differential diagnosis of the weakness to be assessed better. In the patient seen face-to-face whose email diagnosis was wrong, a video clip would almost certainly have enabled the correct diagnosis to be made. Real-time telemedicine seems ideal in theory, but in practice it is likely to be too expensive, time-consuming and difficult to arrange for widespread use. However, it is possible to envisage a triage system in which if email examination was not felt to be diagnostic, then a video clip could be sent; if the diagnosis was still in doubt, then a real-time consultation could be considered. This may be fanciful at present but may become practicable in the future, as broadband communications become available more widely in the developing world.

Thus, as long as neurologists are prepared to accept that they are not always going to get things right, then they can make a difference to patients in the developing world by using email teleneurology. What we have done so far is to deal with the tip of the iceberg. Sorting out the rest will require the efforts of more neurologists and more catalysts, such as the SCT.

Further information

Vassallo DJ. Telemedicine kept simple. www.health.gov.mt/impaedcard/issue/issue3/0116/0116.htm. Accessed 11 February 2005.

References

1. Bergen DC. The world-wide burden of neurologic disease. *Neurology* 1996; **47**: 21–25.
2. Bergen DC. Preventable neurological diseases worldwide. *Neuroepidemiology* 1998; **17**: 67–73.
3. Bergen DC. Training and distribution of neurologists worldwide. *Journal of Neurological Science* 2002; **198**: 3–7.
4. Vassallo DJ, Hoque F, Roberts MF *et al*. An evaluation of the first year's experience with a low-cost telemedicine link in Bangladesh. *Journal of Telemedicine and Telecare* 2001; **7**: 125–138.
5. Graham LE, Zimmerman M, Vassallo DJ *et al*. Telemedicine: the way ahead for medicine in the developing world. *Tropical Doctor* 2003; **33**: 36–38.
6. Hersh D, Hersch F, Mikuletic L, Neilson S. A web-based approach to low-cost telemedicine. *Journal of Telemedicine and Telecare* 2003; **9** (suppl. 2): 24–26.
7. Robib and Telemedicine. Robib Telemedicine Clinic January 2005. www.camnet.com.kh/cambodiaschools/villageleap/telemedicine/Jan_05.htm. Accessed 10 February 2005.
8. Patterson V, Hoque F, Vassallo D *et al*. Store-and-forward teleneurology in developing countries. *Journal of Telemedicine and Telecare* 2001; **7** (suppl. 1): 52-3.
9. Wootton R. Design and implementation of an automatic message-routing system for low-cost telemedicine. *Journal of Telemedicine and Telecare* 2003; **9** (suppl. 1): 44–47.
10. Craig J, Chua R, Russell C *et al*. A cohort study of early neurological consultation by telemedicine on the care of neurological inpatients. *Journal of Neurology, Neurosurgery and Psychiatry* 2004; **75**: 1031–1035.
11. Chua R, Craig J, Wootton R, Patterson V. Randomised controlled trial of telemedicine for new neurological outpatient referrals. *Journal of Neurology, Neurosurgery and Psychiatry* 2001; **71**: 63–66.
12. Craig J, Patterson V, Rocke L, Jamison J. Accident and emergency neurology: time for a reappraisal? *Health Trends* 1997; **3**: 89–91.
13. Patterson V, Humphreys J, Chua R. Email triage of new neurological outpatient referrals from general practice. *Journal of Neurology, Neurosurgery and Psychiatry* 2004; **75**: 617–620.

▶11

Telemedicine in Paediatric Neurology

Anthony C Smith and James T Pelekanos

Introduction

The use of online communication techniques for the delivery of health services to families including children and adolescents has been described in a variety of clinical fields. Apart from our own experience with telepaediatrics in Queensland, the other well-known examples of paediatric telemedicine services are in oncology, cardiology, fetal medicine and psychiatry. Some experience has also been reported in neonatal intensive care for psychosocial support, school-based health-promotion activities, radiology and home care for patient monitoring and support.[1]

Literature review

Despite a growth in the literature on telemedicine, there are few descriptions of the use of online communications in paediatrics. A review of the MEDLINE database (1995–2004) similar to that used by Youngberry[2] and including search terms related to paediatrics and neurology showed very limited evidence of teleneurology in general and only a few papers on paediatric teleneurology (see Table 11.1). Despite pioneering work in adult teleneurology conducted in Northern Ireland,[3–5] there has been little telemedicine work in paediatric neurology. From a collection of 126 articles, we found that 15 had some relevance to paediatrics and only three specifically described work in paediatric teleneurology.

Table 11.1. Number of articles located in the MEDLINE database depending on search term(s) used (1995–January 2004)

Search term(s)	No. of articles
Children or child	1 190 148
Paediatrics or pediatrics	200 855
(Children or child) or (paediatrics or pediatrics)	1 280 206
Telemedicine or telehealth	10 055
(Children or child or paediatrics or pediatrics) and (telemedicine or telehealth)	676
Neurology	199 178
(Children or child or paediatrics or pediatrics) and neurology	29 350
(Telemedicine or telehealth) and neurology	126
(Children or child or paediatrics or pediatrics) and (telemedicine or telehealth) and neurology	15
Telepaediatrics or telepediatrics	4

The first of these described a telephone consulting service in Canada that provided a telephone link between nurse practitioners and specialists.[6] This study addressed the problem of lack of paediatric neurologists and described how a dedicated telephone service staffed by trained nurses helped in the management of patients without physician assistance. Urgent cases that did require physician assistance could be triaged appropriately through the nursing service.

Another type of service was offered by a group in Portugal who developed a neurology teleconsulting network for general practitioners (GPs).[7] This service used low-bandwidth videoconferencing between the GPs and specialists based in the university hospital. During a 12-month period, 88 patients were referred to this service. In this example, teleneurology consultations were very useful for access to specialist advice and for the prevention of unnecessary patient transfers and laboratory tests.

The third study, a US telemedicine service for children with a range of special health needs (including neurology), also reported a high level of satisfaction from staff involved in the service.[8] Evaluation of this programme found that the acceptance of telemedicine by clinicians was more likely to increase with experience.

Websites

Other general reports of paediatric teleneurology were found using the Internet search engine Google (http://google.com/). Websites were located using search terms such as 'neurology', 'telehealth', 'telemedicine', 'teleneurology', 'paediatrics' and 'children'. Most web pages included descriptions of papers or organizational reports related to adult teleneurology services. There was one presentation that described the clinical outcomes of paediatric teleneurology clinics conducted in the USA.[9] This study involved the operation of a routine teleneurology outpatient service for the assessment and/or follow-up of children with neurological conditions, such as epilepsy. According to this report, about 60 consultations were conducted per year. Essentially, the clinicians involved in this service were confident that videoconferencing was an effective method for the diagnosis of new patients with suspected neurological conditions and was valuable for reviewing existing patients.

There were also reports on the Telemedicine Information Exchange database (http://tie.telemed.org/), which listed neurology as a subspecialist area of overall telemedicine programmes. Apart from general summaries, these reports did not tend to describe specific details of activity or results of evaluations, especially in the field of paediatric neurology.

As is evident, there is very little published information about paediatric teleneurology. We describe in more detail our own experience of paediatric teleneurology in Queensland, Australia.

Problems of healthcare delivery in Queensland

Queensland is the second largest state in Australia, with a land area seven times larger than the UK (Fig. 11.1). Queensland is the third most populated state in Australia, with an estimated 3.9 million people.[10] Each year, there are about 50 000 births in

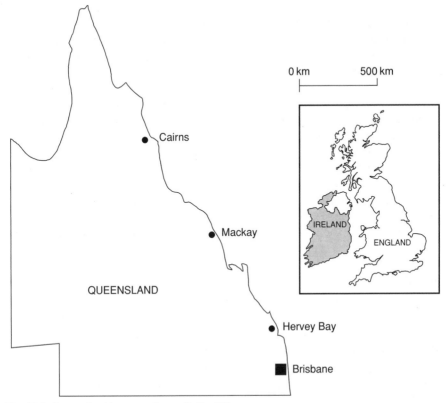

Fig. 11.1. Queensland in comparison with the UK.

Queensland. The Australian Bureau of Statistics (ABS) has predicted that by 2025, the number of children and young people aged 0–24 years will increase by more than 30%.[11] This presents a major challenge for the state health department regarding allocating its resources to children and young people more strategically and cost-effectively than ever before.[12]

Since most specialist health services are situated in the south-east corner of Queensland, the majority of patients who live outside Brisbane must travel or wait for the next outreach clinic if available. In Queensland, the public healthcare system subsidizes the costs of travel for specialist appointments through a patient travel scheme, ie for costs such as airfares, fuel and accommodation. The department also pays for costs associated with the delivery of outreach programmes, where specialists travel out to rural and remote areas for outlying clinics. These costs include travel, accommodation and salaries of the specialists involved. Patient travel schemes and specialist outreach clinics are significant costs to the department. During 2002–03, costs related to patient travel alone for the health department reached AUS$25 million (US$20 million).[13]

Availability of paediatric neurologists is a serious problem. Queensland has only three paediatric neurologists (all based in Brisbane), which in terms of the ratio of specialists to people under the age of 15 years is about one to 260 000, making it the most disadvantaged state in Australia according to a 2003 workforce report conducted by the Royal Australasian College of Physicians (Table 11.2).[14]

Each year, about 1100 outpatient appointments are conducted at the Royal Children's Hospital (RCH) in Brisbane for children who need to be seen by a paediatric neurologist.[15] A substantial proportion of these patients live in non-metropolitan areas and therefore travel significant distances to see a specialist.

We have had over four years' experience in trialling and integrating telemedicine into the routine outpatient services of many paediatric subspecialties, including neurology.

Table 11.2. Number of people under 15 years of age per paediatric neurologist

State	No. of paediatric neurologists	No. of people aged < 15 years per neurologist
Queensland	3	263 000
New South Wales	12	111 000
Western Australia	4	100 000
Victoria	10	96 000
South Australia	3	96 000

Telepaediatrics in Queensland

In November 2000, we established a novel telepaediatric service offering a centralized service to selected sites in Queensland.[16] The aim of the telepaediatric service was to allow staff in outlying areas to make telepaediatric referrals to specialists in Brisbane in the most convenient manner. Outlying hospital staff members were encouraged to refer all queries to a service coordinator. Once a referral was made, the coordinator took full responsibility for managing referrals and guaranteed a response by an appropriate specialist, usually within 24 hours. Responses included returned telephone calls, emails and appointments via videoconference. About 90% of all referrals made to the service resulted in an appointment via videoconference.

Technical requirements

Telepaediatric services were provided from the studios in the Centre for Online Health (COH), situated at the RCH in Brisbane. The studios provide an appropriate environment for telemedicine work, including factors such as room lighting suitable for TV and sound-proofing. In order for telepaediatric activity to take place at the outlying sites, improved videoconferencing facilities were installed and minor room modifications were made. Standard videoconference systems were used (Sony PCS-11, Sony 6000, Tokyo, Japan), as well as peripheral equipment such as a document camera. Videoconferencing was conducted using integrated services digital network

(ISDN) transmission at a preferred minimum bandwidth of 384 kbit/s. Dedicated ISDN lines were installed at each outlying site.

Activity

Since the commencement of the research trial, there has been a steady growth in the number of clinical consultations taking place. The average number of consultations increased from 20 per month in 2000 to about 55 consultations per month in 2004. More than 2000 patient consultations were conducted during the first four years of operation, making it one of the largest telepaediatric services reported in the literature.[16–23] Nonetheless, we estimate that the service is currently reaching only about 20% of the paediatric population in rural and remote areas of Queensland, so the potential for wider expansion is considerable.

A broad range of services has been delivered, comprising over 30 different paediatric subspecialties. The top 15 subspecialties are illustrated in Fig. 11.2. The most common applications have been for post-acute burns care, diabetes, neurology and oncology. Other fields include cardiology, psychiatry, gastroenterology, nephrology and orthopaedics.

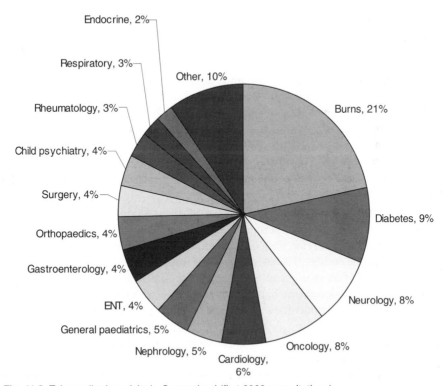

Fig. 11.2. Telepaediatric activity in Queensland (first 2000 consultations).
ENT, ear, nose and throat.

Telemedicine in paediatric neurology

We reviewed our neurology experience within telepaediatrics by examining the hospital records for all patients seen during 2004. The primary diagnosis of each patient, the main purpose of the consultation and the outcome following the videoconference appointment were determined. Information from patient records was also used as the basis for the two case reports mentioned later in this chapter.

Main applications

We used videoconferencing principally for the delivery of clinical services to children living outside the metropolitan area. First and most commonly, videoconferencing was useful for the routine follow-up of patients who required a review by a paediatric neurologist (routine clinics). Second, videoconferencing was valuable for the provision of specialist advice and support to clinicians in remote areas for acute clinical problems. Third, we used videoconferencing for multi-site meetings for case discussions and educational meetings involving specialists based in Brisbane and Cairns (situated about 1700 km north of Brisbane).

Clinical applications

Neurology, like many of the telepaediatric services available through the COH, has become a routine component of the hospital outpatient service. The overall proportion of paediatric neurology consultations increased from 4% (12 consultations) during 2001 to 14% (101 consultations) in 2004 (Fig. 11.3). This substantial growth was probably due to the development of routine weekly videoconference clinics involving two selected paediatric units in Queensland. The majority (94%) of our clinics involved these hospitals in Mackay and Hervey Bay, which are located about 1100 km and 300 km, respectively, from Brisbane. This weekly videoconference clinic gave patients in rural and remote areas of Queensland an opportunity to travel to their local hospital for review by the specialist via videoconference.

Referral process

A critical factor in our programme was that the telepaediatric coordinator from the COH provided full support to both outlying and central staff from the first point of referral. We offered outlying sites convenient access to the coordinator via a single toll-free telephone number. The coordinator was responsible for receiving all referrals and for facilitating an appropriate response by a specialist. If a videoconference was required, then the coordinator liaised between the referring clinician and specialist staff, scheduled the appointment, and provided full technical support during the consultation.

In paediatric neurology, weekly clinics were scheduled 12 months in advance, giving outlying staff the opportunity to plan clinic workloads and make referrals when convenient. Establishing routine clinics also gave the specialist in Brisbane the opportunity to allocate a set time during the week with consideration for any pre-existing hospital commitments. Referrals could be made easily by the local

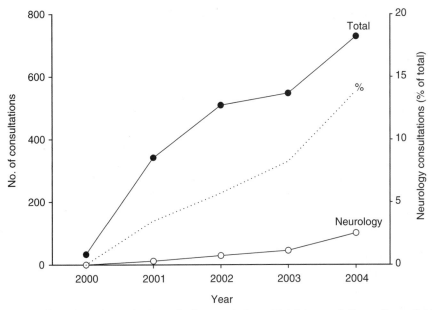

Fig. 11.3. Annual numbers of telepaediatric consultations (● total consultations, ○ paediatric neurology consultations). The dotted line is the proportion of consultations that were paediatric neurology.

paediatrician, who contacted a telepaediatric coordinator with patient details before the clinic. Non-urgent patients were booked into the next available routine clinic; a separate consultation was arranged sooner if a patient was deemed urgent (Fig. 11.4).

As part of the referral process and organization of telepaediatric consultations, a single-page summary sheet (Fig. 11.5) was completed by the referring doctor for each patient and faxed to the COH at least two days before the appointment. The patient summary form was important for several reasons. First, it provided the necessary details for the telepaediatric coordinator to make up a hospital medical record for documentation during the clinic. Second, it provided the specialist with some background information before the clinic, which allowed for the collection of any test results held centrally. Third, the forms helped to expedite the consultation process by prompting referring staff to collate important test results, provide a brief clinical history and clarify the main purpose of the consultation.

Consultation process

At the beginning of each consultation, the referring paediatrician introduced the case (usually without the family present) by outlining the clinical problem and reason for the consultation. The referring doctor next introduced the family to the specialist and then remained an active participant during the consultation. Additional information could also be shared during the videoconference using a document camera.

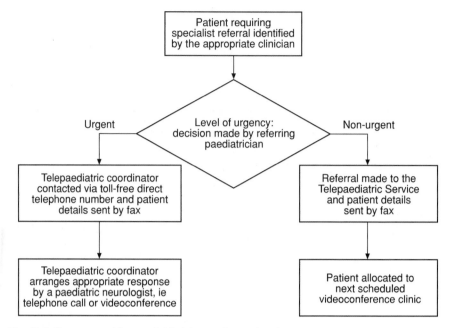

Fig. 11.4. Process used for paediatric teleneurology referrals.

Review of clinical consultations

Since we commenced our work in 2000, we have conducted 187 consultations in the area of paediatric neurology. During 2004, there were 101 consultations on 63 patients at 32 clinics. Thirty-one (49%) of these patients were new referrals; the remaining 32 (51%) were for the follow-up of patients seen previously by the paediatric neurologist.

The patient and family were present in 71 (70%) of these consultations; the remainder involved case discussions, which the patient did not attend (see Figs 11.6 and 11.7). Of the 63 patients who had a paediatric neurology consultation, 56% were female. The age range is shown in Fig. 11.8. Almost half (45%) of all patients seen during 2004 had only one consultation during the 12-month period (Fig. 11.9). Eighteen patients had two consultations. One patient who had a very complex medical history required six consultations for ongoing monitoring and advice regarding his medication regime.

Our weekly videoconference clinics were scheduled to last one hour each. The average duration was actually 56 minutes, with at least three patients seen per clinic.

Diagnosis

Table 11.3 lists the final diagnoses in patients seen during 2004. More than half (54%) of all children referred had the primary diagnosis of epilepsy.

TELEPAEDIATRIC SUMMARY
GENERAL

(Affix Patient Label)

REFERRAL DETAILS	
Referred by:	Hospital / Facility:
Date of videoconference:	
Referred to:	

CONSULTATION DETAILS		
Mother's name:	Father's Name:	Other:
Presenting problem:		
Reason for tele-consultation:		
Relevant history & findings:		
Previous consultation:		
Hospital admissions:		
Investigations:		
Current medication:		
Additional notes:		
Planned presentation:		
☐ Patient present	☐ Video	☐ Photograph
☐ XR / CT	☐ ECHO	☐ PowerPoint
☐ Other staff		

Fig. 11.5. General summary form completed and faxed to specialist before videoconference appointment.

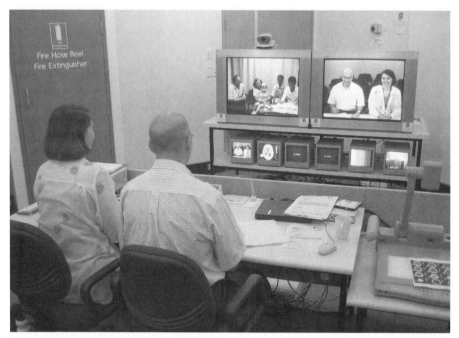

Fig. 11.6. Paediatric neurologist in Brisbane conducting a routine consultation with the patient, family and local paediatrician in Mackay (on screen).

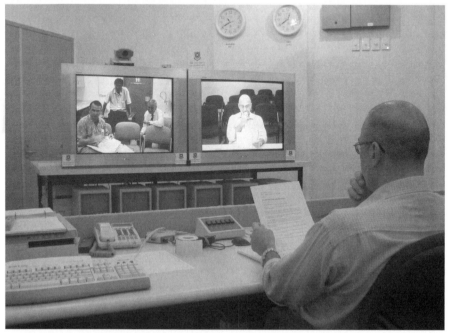

Fig. 11.7. Case discussion between the paediatric neurologist in Brisbane and local paediatricians in Hervey Bay (on screen).

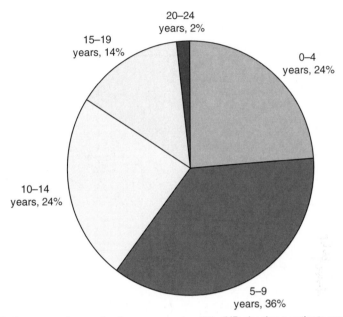

Fig. 11.8. Patients sorted according to age group ($n = 63$). (NB: the three patients aged 19 years and over were followed up by the paediatric neurologist who was responsible for their long-term management.)

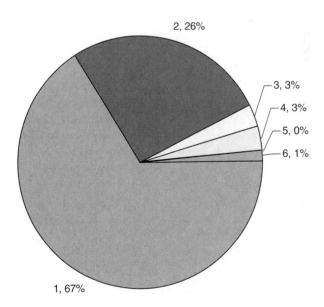

Fig. 11.9. Number of consultations per patient during the 12-month period ($n = 63$).

Table 11.3. Primary diagnosis of patients managed by videoconference during 2004

Primary diagnosis	Number of patients
Epilepsy	34
Tourette's syndrome	5
Absent episodes	5
Headaches	3
Muscle weakness	3
Rett syndrome	2
Autistic spectrum disorder	2
Neurofibromatosis	2
Sturge-Weber syndrome	1
Nocturnal cramps	1
Moyamoya syndrome	1
Mitochondrial disorder	1
Hydrocephalus	1
Conversion disorder	1
Anxiety attacks	1
Total	**63**

Purpose of consultation

Specific reasons for referral to a videoconference included management advice, advice regarding diagnosis, review of medications, discussion of test results and a general case discussion, which often covered most of the above (Fig. 11.10). As described earlier, the majority of patients had chronic health conditions, such as epilepsy, which required intermittent review by a paediatric neurologist. Under normal circumstances, these patients would have travelled to Brisbane to see the specialist in an outpatient clinic.

Outcome of consultation

As shown in Fig. 11.11, a significant proportion of consultations conducted during 2004 resulted in adjustments to medication prescriptions (42%) and recommendations for further tests and investigations (20%). In a few cases, arrangements were made for planned admission or referral to another health professional.

Challenges

The efficient running of a videoconference clinic depends on the interaction between outlying and specialist staff. Consultations were more difficult if the patient was unknown to the local staff member presenting the case. This occurred when the senior paediatrician was unavailable and the case was presented by a resident, who might be unfamiliar with the patient's problems. These consultations took longer than usual.

One problem often reported by critics of videoconferencing is the inability to conduct a physical assessment. However, we were confident with physical assessments performed by the local paediatrician and demonstrations (such as gait)

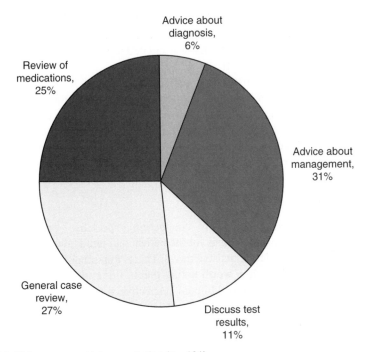

Fig. 11.10. Main purpose of teleconsultation ($n = 101$).

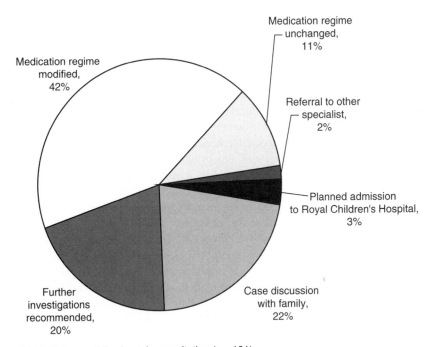

Fig. 11.11. Outcome following teleconsultation ($n = 101$).

shown in full view of the videoconference camera. In our experience, paediatric neurology cases rarely required any physical assessment; the critical aspect of the teleconsultation was the case history that was elicited during the consultation from the patient, family and healthcare staff.

Technical difficulties can affect the smooth running of clinics. Since 2001, we have experienced only two minor technical problems. One was due to the incorrect use of a videoconference system remote control and the other was due to an unexpected ISDN line fault. In the first instance, the problem was rectified by shutting down the videoconference system, rebooting it and re-establishing the videoconference call. In the second instance, we re-established the videoconference call by using a different set of ISDN numbers.

Advantages

There are many advantages of conducting specialist consultations via videoconference. The most obvious is for the patient and family, who are able to see a specialist without the need for extensive travel. This is important since the distances in Queensland are very large. It is worth noting that to drive to Brisbane from Hervey Bay or Mackay takes about four or 11 hours, respectively. A recent study examined the costs and time involved in attending an outpatient appointment in person at the RCH or via videoconference through our telepaediatric service; 400 families were interviewed. There were significant differences between the two groups. Families who could travel to their local hospital for a videoconference appointment reported much less inconvenience and significantly less expense than those families that travelled to Brisbane for their appointment.[22]

Videoconferencing also allowed for the screening of patients, ensuring that only those patients who definitely required admission to the RCH were actually transferred. If transfer was considered appropriate, then mechanisms were put in place for the coordination of the admission, including the scheduling of appointments with other specialists and the booking of hospital investigations.

For many of the other subspecialist services we offer through the telepaediatric service, there has been a reduction in the number of physical outreach visits conducted by specialists based in Brisbane. Videoconference clinics have been arranged to complement annual outreach visits. We have found this to be the best approach to the delivery of specialist services in rural areas, especially when large distances are involved.[24] Unfortunately, in paediatric neurology, due to the limited number of specialists, physical outreach clinics do not occur. Videoconferencing in this context therefore is an excellent alternative for contact with clinicians and patients in outlying centres.

From the perspective of the outlying hospitals, the involvement of the local staff responsible for the care of the patient enables the promotion of local case management and coordination of services in close proximity to the patient. The other key advantage is related to educational opportunities for staff involved in the videoconference. By participating in the consultation, both senior and junior staff members in the referring hospitals have the opportunity to discuss complex cases and the rationale behind chosen treatment regimes. Normally, this type of interaction does not occur because once a patient is transferred to the RCH, he or she is reviewed independently by the specialist. In the latter case, communication between the referring doctor and specialist was mainly by referral letters and reports sent back by the specialist.

Case report 1: management of complex cases via videoconference

CM was a 14-year-old female with epilepsy, intellectual impairment and behavioural difficulties. Her epilepsy began at four months of age and had been refractory to treatment with all known antiepileptic medications. Eighteen months earlier, she had a vagal nerve stimulator (VNS) implanted, which resulted in a moderate decrease in the severity of her seizures. CM had undergone extensive investigations, including neuro-imaging and metabolic tests, which failed to identify an aetiology for her condition. In the past, the family had to travel on numerous occasions from Mackay to Brisbane for appropriate specialist treatment.

CM was seen in a videoconference clinic twice in 2004. On the first occasion, her medications were adjusted. On the second occasion, a number of other issues were raised and it was decided that CM should again come to Brisbane for further investigations. This included a repeat magnetic resonance imaging (MRI) scan. The VNS needed to be turned off for this procedure, and the computer system required this to be booked in advance. CM also underwent a positron-emission tomography (PET) scan, which did not reveal any focal lesions, therefore excluding the possibility of epilepsy surgery. Finally, she had episodic altered behaviour. On clinical grounds, it was not certain whether this was seizure-related or part of her behavioural disorder. A 24-hour video electroencephalography (EEG) study confirmed that it was seizure-related. Further trials of medications were undertaken.

This case raises extremely difficult and complex medical and social problems. The benefits of videoconferencing in this context include a reduction in the amount of travel to Brisbane required, better pre-admission planning (ie more efficient coordination of complex investigations), and improved communication between the family, local paediatrician and paediatric neurologists.

Case report 2: diagnosis and treatment of a child with Tourette's syndrome

KS was a nine-year-old girl diagnosed with Tourette's syndrome. She began experiencing multifocal motor and vocal tics at 6.5 years of age. As well as tics, people with Tourette's syndrome often have one or more comorbid features, including attention deficit hyperactivity disorder (ADHD) and obsessive compulsive disorder (OCD).[25] These comorbid features often are clinically more important than the tic disorder. In this case, detailed history-taking during the teleconsultation revealed a number of obsessive and ritualistic features that were interfering with the patient's school and social activities. These OCD symptoms were treated with sertraline; at follow-up four months later, her level of functioning had improved markedly.

This case demonstrates how an initial consultation via videoconference allowed for the accurate identification and treatment of core difficulties in a patient with Tourette's syndrome. Additionally, there were educational benefits, as the general paediatricians who participated in this consultation subsequently identified and treated several other similar patients locally.

Educational applications

In addition to the clinical consultations that we have conducted via videoconference, we have also used videoconferencing for the delivery of a series of interactive meetings related to the management of epilepsy. These meetings serve as an interactive forum between specialists in Brisbane and Cairns to discuss a broad range of issues associated with epilepsy. Discussion topics so far have included the surgical approach to patients with complex focal epilepsy, seizure localization, antiepileptic medication use, and practical issues in delivering services to patients with epilepsy.

During 2004, six sessions, each lasting about 90 minutes, were coordinated. On average, there were 15 participants in Brisbane and three participants in Cairns. Originally meetings were held in the COH via videoconference at a bandwidth of 384 kbit/s. Due to a growing number of participants, these meetings were relocated to a larger venue within the hospital. Unfortunately, there were some difficulties making a 384 kbit/s call at this venue, so we had to settle for a low-speed connection of 128 kbit/s. We found that the higher bandwidth was essential for the interpretation of video EEG. In cases where bandwidth was low, there were difficulties in recognizing important aspects of the video recordings. Apart from the real-time video recordings, all other aspects worked extremely well. Sessions were semi-structured in workshop format, allowing for the presentation of material using PowerPoint slides and picture-archiving and communications systems (PACS) via the local hospital network for the transmission of recorded video EEG data. All sites were able to share their experiences and opinions related to this specialist area (Fig. 11.12).

Case report 3: Epilepsy Interest Group discussions via videoconference

MH is a 15-year-old boy with refractory epilepsy and mild intellectual difficulties. He was born with cyanotic congenital heart disease and suffered a right cerebral hemisphere stroke in the first week of life. MH has a complete left hemiplegia and hemianopia. His current neuro-imaging shows a complete infarction of the right middle cerebral artery territory. He had some initial seizures in the neonatal period but then he was seizure-free until four years of age, at which time the seizures recurred and have not responded to numerous antiepileptic medications. The details of this case, including the semiology of the seizures and the patient's neuro-imaging and ictal video EEG studies, were discussed by the members of the Epilepsy Interest Group. The

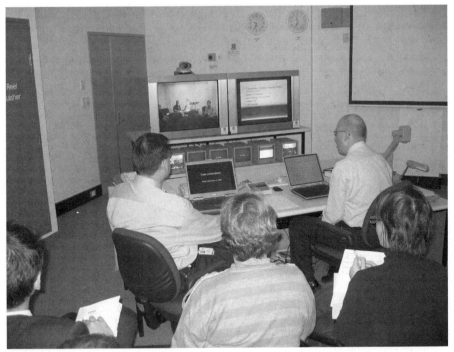

Fig. 11.12. Videoconference epilepsy meetings involving specialists in Brisbane and Cairns (on screen).

consensus of the meeting was that there was enough evidence to proceed with further investigations, with a view to performing epilepsy surgery.

Conclusion

Telemedicine can be applied usefully to paediatric neurology. Paediatric teleneurology has the advantage over its adult counterpart of not being dependent on a detailed neurological examination, and this should make its more widespread introduction easier. The system we used is clearly feasible and is acceptable to patients and users. It is effective in providing acutely admitted patients with prompt management advice and reduces the costs associated with patient travel to a specialist hospital and unnecessary hospital admission. It also has considerable educational aspects, both informal and formal, both for consultants and for doctors in training at outlying hospitals.

The model of service delivery that we use is based on the involvement of a telehealth coordinator, and the advantages of this are considerable. Specifically, it reduces any reticence or technological phobia on the part of doctors about videoconferencing by making the technical aspects of the consultation the responsibility of the coordinator. All the doctor has to do is to concentrate on diagnosis and management of the patient. The virtual absence of technical problems then fosters increasing medical confidence in the system. Telemedicine currently is being used in paediatric neurology in only a few places in the world, and yet people in many areas are likely to benefit from such a service. We hope that the information provided here will help to support the development of similar paediatric teleneurology services, especially in areas where large distances cause isolation between the specialist and patient.

Acknowledgements

The Telepaediatric Service is funded by the Commonwealth Department of Health and Ageing (Medical Specialist Outreach Assistance Programme).

Further information

The International Child Neurology Association is a non-profit-making association of child neurologists and members of allied professions from all parts of the world dedicated to promoting clinical and scientific research in the field of child neurology and encouraging the recognition of child neurologist's competence and scope of practice: www.child-neuro.net/. Accessed 27 January 2005.

The Child Neurology Association is a non-profit-making professional association of paediatric neurologists in the USA, Canada and worldwide devoted to fostering the discipline of child neurology and promoting the optimum care and welfare of children with neurological and neurodevelopmental disorders. These disorders include epilepsy, cerebral palsy, mental retardation, learning disabilities, complex metabolic diseases, nerve and muscle diseases and other highly challenging conditions: www.childneurologysociety.org/. Accessed 27 January 2005.

The Child Neurology Home Page coordinates the available Internet resources in child neurology, for both professionals and patients: www-personal.umich.edu/~leber/c-n/. Accessed 27 January 2005.

References

1 Wootton R, Batch J. *Telepediatrics: Telemedicine and Child Health*. London: Royal Society of Medicine Press, 2005.
2 Youngberry K. Telemedicine research and MEDLINE. *Journal of Telemedicine and Telecare* 2004; **10**: 121–123.
3 Patterson V. Teleneurology in Northern Ireland: a success. *Journal of Telemedicine and Telecare* 2002; **8** (suppl. 3): 46–47.
4 Chua R, Craig J, Esmonde T *et al*. Telemedicine for new neurological outpatients: putting a randomized controlled trial in the context of everyday practice. *Journal of Telemedicine and Telecare* 2002; **8**: 270–273.
5 Craig J, Chua R, Russell C *et al*. A cohort study of early neurological consultation by telemedicine on the care of neurological inpatients. *Journal of Neurology, Neurosurgery and Psychiatry* 2004; **75**: 1031–1035.

6 Kempe A, Dempsey C, Whitefield J *et al*. Appropriateness of urgent referrals by nurses at a hospital-based pediatric call center. *Archives of Pediatric and Adolescent Medicine* 2000; **154**: 355–360.

7 Paiva T, Coelho H, Araujo MT *et al*. Neurological teleconsultation for general practitioners. *Journal of Telemedicine and Telecare* 2001; **7**: 149–154.

8 Karp WB, Grigsby RK, McSwiggan-Hardin M *et al*. Use of telemedicine for children with special health care needs. *Pediatrics* 2000; **105**: 843–847.

9 Niesen C, Riley R, Klee M *et al*. Clinical Outcome in a Pediatric Teleneurology Clinic. www.atmeda.org/news/2003_presentations/T2e1.niesen.htm. Accessed 25 January 2005.

10 Australian Bureau of Statistics. Australian Demographic Statistics. Catalogue no. 3101.0. www.abs.gov.au/Ausstats/abs%40.nsf/e8ae5488b598839cca25682000131612/6949409dc8b8fb92ca25 6bc60001b3d1!OpenDocument. Accessed 25 January 2005.

11 Australian Bureau of Statistics. Population Growth: Australia's Child Population. 1997, Catalogue no. 3222.0. www.abs.gov.au. Accessed 25 January 2005.

12 Queensland Health. *A Strategic Policy Framework for Children and Young People's Health 2002–2007*. Brisbane: Child and Youth Health Unit, 2002.

13 Queensland Health. *Queensland Health Annual Report 2002–2003*. Brisbane: Queensland Government, 2003.

14 Royal Australasian College of Physicians. *Clinical Workforce in Internal Medicine and Paediatrics in Australasia 2003*. Sydney: Royal Australasian College of Physicians, 2004.

15 Royal Children's Hospital Foundation. *Royal Children's Hospital Foundation Queensland, Annual Report, 2003*. Brisbane: Royal Children's Hospital, 2003.

16 Smith AC, Isles A, McCrossin R *et al*. The point-of-referral barrier: a factor in the success of telehealth. *Journal of Telemedicine and Telecare* 2001; **7** (suppl. 2): 75–78.

17 Smith AC, Youngberry K, Mill J *et al*. A review of three years experience using email and videoconferencing for the delivery of post-acute burns care to children in Queensland. *Burns* 2004: **30**: 248–252.

18 Smith AC, Williams M, Justo R. The multidisciplinary management of a paediatric cardiac emergency. *Journal of Telemedicine and Telecare* 2002; **8**: 112–114.

19 Smith AC, Kairl JA, Kimble R. Post-acute care for a paediatric burns patient in regional Queensland. *Journal of Telemedicine and Telecare* 2002; **8**: 302–304.

20 Smith AC, Williams M, Van Der Westhuyzen J *et al*. A comparison of telepaediatric activity at two regional hospitals in Queensland. *Journal of Telemedicine and Telecare* 2002; **8** (suppl. 3): 58–62.

21 Smith AC, Batch J, Lang E, Wootton R. The use of online health techniques to assist with the delivery of specialist paediatric diabetes services in Queensland. *Journal of Telemedicine and Telecare* 2003; **9** (suppl. 2): 54–57.

22 Smith AC, Youngberry K, Christie F *et al*. The family costs of attending hospital outpatient appointments via videoconference and in person. *Journal of Telemedicine and Telecare* 2003; **9** (suppl. 2): 58–61.

23 Justo R, Smith AC, Williams M *et al*. Paediatric telecardiology services in Queensland: a review of three years' experience. *Journal of Telemedicine and Telecare* 2004; **10** (suppl. 2): 57–60.

24 Williams M, Smith AC. Paediatric outreach services. *Journal of Paediatrics and Child Health* 2004; **40**: 501–503.

25 Jankovic J. Tourette's syndrome. *New England Journal of Medicine* 2001. **345**: 1184–1192.

Section 3: Practical Issues

▶12

How to do a Real-Time Teleneurology Examination

Victor Patterson, Danny McArdle and Sinead Gormley

Introduction

The process of a real-time teleneurology consultation is relatively straightforward, but there are a few traps for the unwary. The failure of a video-consultation saps the confidence of patients and users alike. Following the advice in this chapter will make failure unlikely and ensure that the neurological teleconsultation is a pleasant experience for everyone concerned.

Equipment and maintenance

Equipment and its maintenance are issues that are linked inextricably.

Equipment

There are a number of well-known manufacturers of videoconferencing equipment, including Tandberg (Lysaker, Norway), Polycom (Pleasanton, USA), Sony (Tokyo, Japan) and Aethra (Aneona, Italy). They make a range of equipment of different complexities and prices. In general, mid-range equipment, eg the Tandberg 880 (Fig. 12.1), is suitable for teleneurology. Desktop equipment, eg the Tandberg 1000

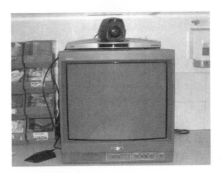

Fig. 12.1. Tandberg 880 on top of a monitor in a ward.

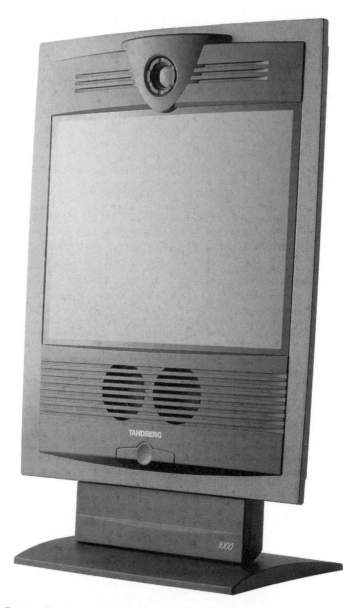

Fig. 12.2. Desktop Tandberg 1000. Note the small built-in camera.

(Fig. 12.2), although superficially attractive, does not have a camera that will transmit a sufficiently good picture of the neurologist or patient. The following properties are important:

▶ *Transmission mode*. Although at present most teleneurology is carried out over an integrated services digital network (ISDN), it is likely that the Internet will become used more widely for telemedicine. Therefore, it is prudent to buy equipment that is capable of both ISDN and Internet Protocol (IP) transmission.

▶ *Pan, tilt and zoom camera.* The quality of the transmitted image is dependent on the camera quality. For a teleneurology examination, the camera needs to have a good range of pan, tilt and zoom, so try them out before buying.

▶ *Robustness.* In clinical situations, knocks are likely to occur and delicate equipment is unlikely to last.

▶ *Far-end control and presets.* Control of the remote camera is essential in a teleneurology examination, as are preset camera positions. It is also important that the preset positions are easy to access during a consultation. This varies greatly with different models, so try it out before buying.

▶ *Encryption.* Data encryption is desirable but probably not essential.

Maintenance

Videoconferencing equipment requires no regular maintenance, but if it is located in a dusty area, then it should be kept covered. Technical breakdowns are dealt with below.

The vendor

Choosing a vendor is rarely considered at the early stages of acquiring videoconferencing equipment. However, the choice of vendor is a crucial decision that should be made as early as possible. Your relationship with the vendor can have a long-term effect on the benefit or cost to your network and could, ultimately, lead to project failure if careful attention is not given to this decision. You should scrutinize a range of different manufacturers' equipment and vendors and see which system best fits your needs and budget.

A good vendor should offer a choice of different manufacturers' equipment. It is important that your chosen vendor has a sound financial profile and company history as well as proven customer service and support. Ask vendors for details of satisfied customers and contact them to enquire about the claims that the vendor is making. Ask for a live demonstration of the videoconferencing equipment, using the communication network of your choice. Are the audio and video qualities good enough to support your needs? Use the equipment and satisfy yourself that you are comfortable with it. What commitment to technical support does the vendor offer if problems arise, eg unlimited access to telephone/video helpline? The vendor should offer delivery, installation and initial training of equipment as part of the purchase price.

Most vendors will offer extended services, at a cost, after the normal equipment manufacturer warranty has ended. These extended service contracts can offer different levels of support and should be agreed with the supplier of the equipment at the time of purchase to cover system failure. The service contracts should include any future system software upgrades and collection and replacement of faulty equipment within an agreed time to reduce system downtime. Maintenance contracts can be expensive overall, so it is important that careful consideration is given to them, otherwise you could be left with a failed project and a lot of expensive unused equipment. Remember: buyer beware![1,2]

Setting up a room at the referring site

Rooms at the centre and at the referring site have different requirements, since a patient will need to be examined at the latter but not at the former.

Location

The most important consideration at the referring site is to choose a room that will be convenient for staff and patients at the referring hospital. Staff members are usually busy, and taking a patient to a telemedicine room can easily be seen as an additional chore. If this process is complicated, then local staff members will find plenty of plausible reasons not to use telemedicine.

To enable local access sometimes requires working in less than ideal circumstances, but proximity should always be the most important consideration. For acute neurology, we use side-rooms adjacent to the ward that are also used for other purposes. The equipment can be either concealed in a cupboard or put on a trolley in the room out of the way (Fig. 12.3).

(a)

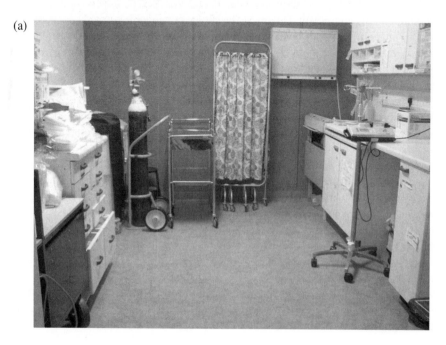

(b)

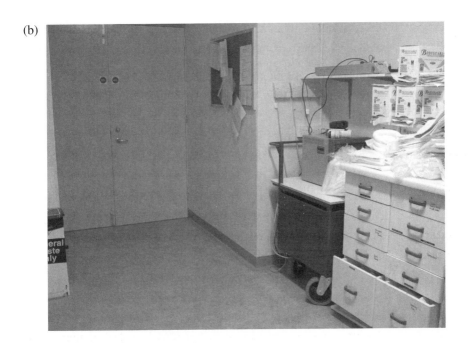

(c)

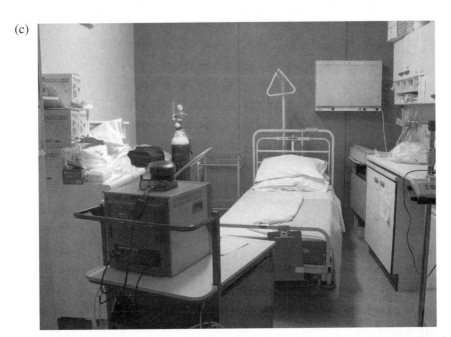

Fig. 12.3. (a) Ward side-room in regular use. (b) Storage of equipment on a purpose-built trolley. (c) Bed in room and equipment in position of use.

Acoustics and lighting

Microphones of videoconferencing equipment are very effective, but sound quality can be improved further by using a room with non-reflective ceilings and carpet. These may be difficult to achieve in a hospital environment. Intermittent distractions such as ice-making machines should be switched off for the duration of the consultation. Natural sunlight makes everybody feel better, and much of the conference can be done under such conditions, but it is important to have a controlled, artificially lit option as well. Major[3] has discussed room design in more detail.

Privacy

If it is not possible to be the only user of the room, then it is important to have a curtained-off area to maintain privacy. A 'Do not disturb' sign on the door may help.

Access

The room should usually contain an examination couch, which will be used for most patients, but it must be possible to replace this with a bed or wheelchair for bed- or wheelchair-bound patients. The door therefore needs to be wide enough to allow access for a bed. There should be space in the room for the camera to capture the patient taking four or five steps to allow assessment of gait.

Colour

A plain colour on the walls, neither too dark nor too bright, is ideal for videoconferencing. We use a light- to mid-blue colour; neutral grey is also a good colour. As far as possible, the background behind the patient should be as plain and homogeneous as possible. Take down any notices and try to have a uniform colour; we repainted our brown-varnished drug cupboard matt blue to achieve this (Fig. 12.4).

Cabling

Once you have decided where the equipment is going and where the patient will be, then it is best to have the necessary telephone lines and power outlets located so that there are no trailing wires.

Positioning everything

Because preset camera positions are used to make the neurological examination shorter, it is necessary to fix both the camera and the bed so that the presets capture the required view every time. This can be done with the aid of marks on the floor or wall for the bed. If the camera is located on top of a monitor on a trolley, then it will be necessary to mark the positions of the camera on the monitor, the monitor on the trolley, and the trolley on the floor.

Viewing X-ray films

To visualize an X-ray film requires either a document camera or a viewing box. We use the latter, focusing the camera on the box using a camera preset. This is because most

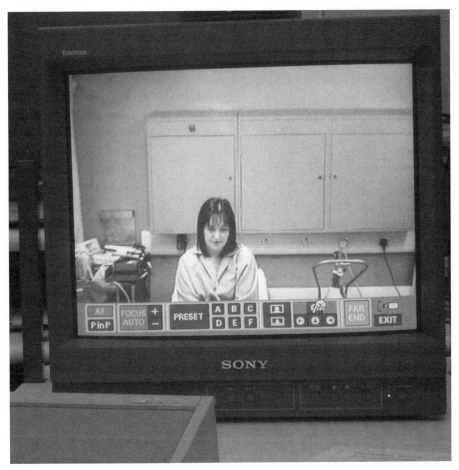

Fig. 12.4. Patient viewed against a near-uniform background.

examination rooms already have a viewing box and may not have enough space for a document camera.

Neurological equipment

The limited equipment necessary to conduct a neurological examination needs to be available easily and constantly to the examining doctor. There are few things more irritating than having to wait while a doctor goes off to search the hospital for a patella hammer.

Setting up the room at the centre

The room to be used by the neurologist can be a purpose-designed studio or an office, or it can even be at the doctor's home. There are advantages and disadvantages to all of these. A studio will usually be better technically and have associated systems designed for telemedicine, with optimal lighting, sound and equipment (Fig. 12.5). It may however, be in a remote part of the hospital, which may discourage use by busy clinicians. Therefore, setting up equipment in a doctor's office may be preferable. With equipment at home, time otherwise spent travelling to hospital may be better used.

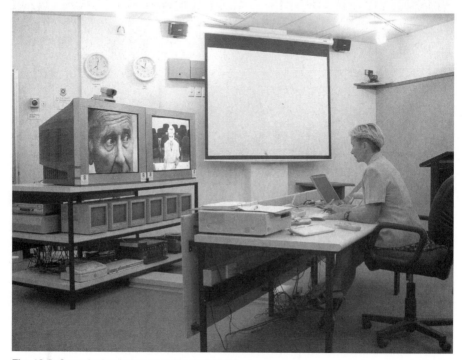

Fig. 12.5. Consultation from a purpose-built studio.

Acoustics

It is important that the doctor and patient can hear each other well. Low ceilings and carpets help, and sound-absorbing walls are also useful. However, although they make the consultation easier, none of these is essential. Telephones (landline and mobile) should be muted, just as they should for conventional consultations.

Vision

The doctor should see the required view of the patient on the whole monitor. At the doctor's end a view of the doctor can be seen either on a separate part of a double monitor (usually in a studio) or as a picture-in-picture in an office. At the patient's end a 'newsreader' view (Fig. 12.6) is best. The doctor's head should be about 10% of the

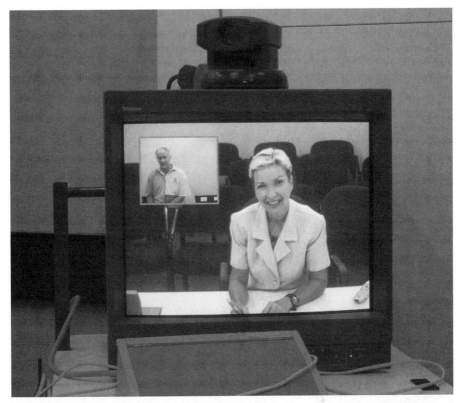

Fig. 12.6. View of neurologist from patient's end. The picture within the picture (top left of screen) shows the patient.

monitor height from the top, and the camera should be positioned on top of the monitor in the centre. When the doctor looks at the patient on the screen, and vice versa, they will then make reasonable eye contact. The background should be uniform, but 'homely' touches such as flowers on the desk are perfectly acceptable (although not yet tested in a randomized controlled trial). In office and home situations, where there is outside light, the brightness of the neurologist may fluctuate with cloud conditions. If the use of artificial light is not an option, then the brightness levels for the neurologist's camera need to be altered; this can be done most easily by having the camera presets on the neurologist's camera set to different levels of brightness.

Communications

During or following a consultation, it is often necessary to send or obtain information, so communication equipment is essential, including a telephone to obtain corroborative history, a fax machine and email to send or receive reports, and a personal computer (PC) with an Internet connection to obtain relevant images by linking to picture-archiving and communication systems (PACS) or radiology web servers. The availability of a telemedicine coordinator in an adjacent room makes this process much easier.

Training

There are three groups of staff members for whom training is important:

Ward and outpatient staff

These staff members will come into contact with the service and the equipment, and so they need some knowledge of what the system is used for, how it works and how to work it if necessary. This information can be conveyed either at occasional formal training sessions or by informal individual or small-group sessions.

Medical staff

These members of staff will be responsible for presenting the patients, so they need to know how to set up the machine, how to dial through to the neurologist, and some simple troubleshooting measures if things go wrong. They do not need to know much about camera control, because this will be done by the neurologist.

In addition, they need to know how to examine the neurological system when a camera is on them. This is the most challenging part of real-time teleneurology. It is apparent that many junior doctors are very poor at examining the nervous system, even when a camera is not present, presumably reflecting the pressure of the medical undergraduate curriculum worldwide. We provide each new group of doctors at each site with a face-to-face training session covering both technical and examination aspects. This has to be repeated twice a year at each site, and this frequency is likely to increase in the future as the curriculum for doctors in training changes. Reinforcement and continuing education are given during patient presentations, but inexpert examination technique undoubtedly slows down the consultation process.

Specialist teleneurology assistants

One solution to the transient nature of junior medical staff is to use nursing assistants to present patients. This requires substantial training in four areas: neurological diseases and their management, practical neurological examination, technical aspects of videoconferencing, and presentation of neurological patients over a videolink. We have developed this training ourselves, and it takes about six months to complete on a part-time basis. Currently, teleneurology assistants present outpatients reliably and effectively (Fig. 12.7),[4] and we are about to extend this method to inpatients. Healthcare organizations need to adapt to this change in service provision and recognize the specialist teleneurology assistants' contributions financially.

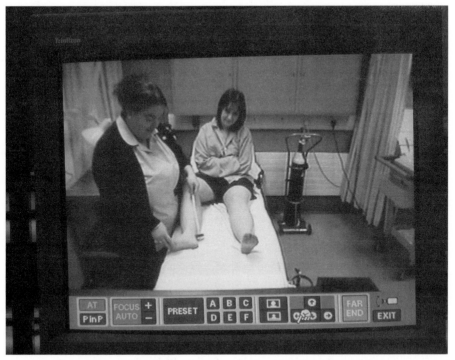

Fig. 12.7. Teleneurology assistant in Omagh (Northern Ireland) eliciting ankle jerks for the neurologist in Brisbane (Australia), approximately 17 000 km away.

Troubleshooting

After initial training, a troubleshooting checklist (Table 12.1) should be attached to each videoconferencing system to enable local staff to deal with basic problems. The troubleshooting protocol will minimize any basic technical problems with the system. Staff can be given a troubleshooting checklist to go through before calling technical support. Telephone contact details of a technician based at the specialist site must be available in case there are problems that cannot be dealt with by staff locally. For example, staff at the remote site may be unable to see an image on their monitor or hear the audio from the specialist due to cables being disconnected accidentally; the technician can instruct remote staff members in how to reconnect the cables via telephone. More advanced problems such as network communication failure can also be diagnosed by telephone.

The failure of the communication network is usually a telephone-company transmission problem rather than a system failure. If this cannot be fixed immediately, then the videoconference may need to be rescheduled for the following day. The importance of having immediate and reliable telephone technical support cannot be

Table 12.1. Troubleshooting checklist

Problem	Cause	Solution
Cannot connect to remote party	Unit is not connected to ISDN line	Connect to ISDN line
	Remote party has not been registered on system	Register remote party
	Remote system is not turned on	Ask the remote party to turn on system
No audio	Cables disconnected	Reconnect cables
	Volume too low	Turn up the volume
	Remote party has muted the sound	Un-mute the sound
	Audio unit is not connected	Connect the audio unit
No video	Cables disconnected	Reconnect cables
	Incorrect camera input	Select main camera
Picture is blurred	Manual focus selected but picture remains blurred	Adjust focus
Transmitted image is dark	Manual brightness is selected	Select auto brightness

ISDN, integrated services digital network.

stressed enough. Most rural hospitals need to go outside of their organization for technical support, as they have little experience in maintaining videoconferencing and network systems to provide a reliable service. Access to telephone support provides reassurance to staff at remote sites and reduces system downtime. Clinical staff will not make use of videoconferencing systems unless such systems can be shown to be reliable and user-friendly.

Pre-examination explanation

Explanations must be provided to two groups of patients before a teleneurology examination can take place:

▶ *Acute inpatients.* Patients are selected for teleneurology consultations by a consultant physician or resident, who will explain what is involved. The nursing staff will explain further, and a laminated patient information sheet is also provided. We do not require patients to sign a written consent form because we consider real-time teleneurology to be routine practice, just as we do not require patients to sign a written consent form before a face-to-face examination.

▶ *Outpatients.* The patient receives a letter giving a time and date for the appointment and stating that this will be a videoconsultation. A telephone number is given to request further information. When the patient arrives, he or she is greeted by the teleneurology assistant, who explains that the consultation will be by videolink, that it will be private and secure, and that the neurologist will introduce anyone with him or her. The patient is asked to change into shorts to facilitate the examination. A laminated information sheet is given to the patient, who is encouraged to ask the assistant any other questions that they may have regarding the consultation.

Setting up the consultation

Booking a consultation

For outpatients, the teleneurology clinic runs identically to its conventional equivalent, with each patient having a pre-arranged appointment time and with a list of patients with their details and referral letters being available to the neurologist.

For an acute neurology service, the situation is more complex because the demand is variable and unpredictable and because multiple hospitals are served and will compete for time slots. The referring doctor contacts the teleneurology coordinator, who allocates a time and location for that doctor to place a video-call to the neurologist.

Transferring information

Before the consultation starts, it is important that the neurologist has the background information about the patient. When the request for the consultation is made, the teleneurology coordinator will record the patient's name, hospital unit number, date of birth and date of admission, and the name of the presenting doctor or nurse. This information will be available to the neurologist at the start of the consultation.

Starting the consultation

When the presenting doctor or nurse dials through, the patient may or may not be present. Our preference is to initiate outpatient consultations without the patient, but for inpatient consultations to have the patient present. If the patient is present, then the general introduction at the start of the next section should be gone through. Anybody accompanying the patient should be positioned beside the patient so that they can all be seen on the screen.

For outpatient consultations the reason for referral should be clear from the correspondence, but for acute referrals the presenting doctor should outline the presentation. For both groups, it is then necessary to obtain the information given in Table 12.2.

The information on previous illness is usually available from the notes, which, unfortunately, are rarely in electronic format. Thus, the first problem is to find what is relevant and the second is to relay it to the neurologist. This can be done either by reading out the information or by placing the relevant page on a document camera or X-ray viewing box. All of these methods are laborious and unquestionably add time to

Table 12.2. Essential information needed before the consultation

History	Previous history
	Previous neurological history
	Current medications
Examination	Temperature, pulse, blood pressure
	Optic fundi
Investigations	Results of those to date

the consultation. They are, however, extremely important, with previous neurological history being especially relevant. Information on the appearance of the optic fundi is important, since during a videoconference these cannot be seen without a dedicated fundus camera.

Taking the history

At the start, the neurologist should greet the patient, introduce him- or herself, and introduce anyone else in the room with them. The neurologist should explain that there is a slight delay in hearing speech, which everybody gets used to quickly. Then it is a matter of letting the patient give the history, with help from any accompanying people if necessary. The camera at the referring end, which the neurologist controls, should be on the patient's face to pick up facial expressions; the patient should see a 'newsreader view' (Fig. 12.6) of the neurologist, with a picture-in-picture showing how they appear to the neurologist. This is also the best camera position in which to examine higher mental functions, which can be done seamlessly at the end of the history-taking.

Interestingly, patients tend to keep more to the point during a teleconsultation than when seen face-to-face, perhaps because of the need to concentrate. The neurologist can write notes during the consultation.

Corroborative history

Corroborative history is essential for patients in coma or with intermittent loss of consciousness or awareness. It is also extremely useful when the patient's history is vague or the diagnosis is unclear. A witness who accompanies the patient is ideal, but if not they can be contacted by telephone at some stage during the consultation, with the microphone being muted at the examiner's end. The widespread availability of mobile phones has greatly reduced the number of failed contacts in this regard.

Performing the examination

Camera presets

A core neurological examination is performed, but in a different sequence to the conventional neurological examination. This is to minimize camera adjustments, which are time-consuming, by using the preset settings on the camera. These enable the neurologist to set the pan, tilt and zoom at the patient's end, together with the light intensity. The latter cannot be set remotely during the examination and must be set at the patient's end; it is especially relevant to examination of the pupils and eye movement, where a high light intensity is required. The neurologist can then move between preset positions at the patient's end by a single click. The examinations at each preset are shown in Table 12.3.

Table 12.3. Preset camera positions for the core teleneurology examination

Preset position				
A	B	C	D	E
Pupils	Arm power	Visual fields	Plantars	Gait
	deltoids			
	finger abductors			
	*biceps/triceps/wrists			
Eye movements	Arm reflexes	Finger–nose test		
Eyelid closure	Leg reflexes	Neck movements		
Mouth closure	Heel–shin test	Truncal stability		
Tongue movements	Arm and leg sensation	Leg power:		
		hip flexors		
		ankle dorsiflexors		
		*knee flexors/extensors		
Palate movement	*Neck stiffness			
*Corneal reflex	*Kernig's sign			
*Facial sensation	Tone			
	Tremor			

*Additional signs.

Additional examinations

It is necessary sometimes to examine additional aspects of neurological function, and suitable viewing angles can be added to the suitable camera preset positions; some of these are marked in Table 12.3 with an asterisk.

Special circumstances

Comatose patients cannot be examined with fixed preset positions. We usually examine such patients in bed in the semi-reclining position, which allows assessment of eye movements and relative limb power, turning the bed through 90 degrees to assess the plantar responses. Profoundly disabled wheelchair-bound patients for whom transfer to a bed would be difficult can have much of the examination performed in a wheelchair, with the neurologist controlling the camera remotely.

Viewing radiological images

It is essential to view computed tomography (CT) and magnetic resonance (MR) images of patients seen, and there are a number of ways in which this can be done. Where a PACS system exists, a separate PACS viewer in the same or adjacent room as the neurologist is ideal. Local web servers also allow this to be done, and the quality is appropriate for assessment by a neurologist. It is also easy to enter into discussion with either the local radiologist or a regional neuroradiologist if necessary. The disadvantages of such a system are that it requires specialized equipment and that it may only operate behind a firewall and so may not be accessible from outside a hospital environment, which makes consulting from home or office difficult. See Chapter 8 for further information.

A less elegant solution is to place the hard copies of the films on a document camera or viewing box in the patient's room. With this technique, we use a preset camera position to focus on the wall-mounted viewing box; we find this easier than using a document camera, which requires someone else to move the films. Although the image is not as good as that seen on a web server, it is usually adequate in the clinical context and where the report of a radiologist is also available (Fig. 12.8).

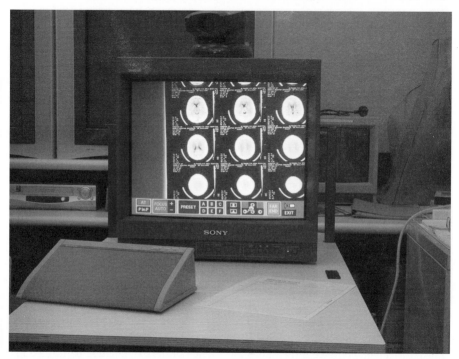

Fig. 12.8. Computed tomography scan film on a viewing box with the patient, seen at the neurologist's end.

Discussion with the patient

As with face-to-face encounters, discussion with the patient is probably the most important part of the consultation. Each doctor will have their own approach. Our usual practice is to tell the patient what we think is causing their symptoms and what we are confident is not. We then go on to talk about necessary tests, treatment and further appointments. It is critically important that the doctor or nurse with the patient is paying close attention to this, as the patient will almost certainly ask them questions after the neurologist has disconnected. The patient then has an opportunity to raise questions, seek clarification or just disagree. If there are accompanying people, they too can be asked if they have any questions.

This process is identical to a face-to-face consultation. Over a videolink it seems more formal, because both parties have to concentrate a little harder. Following a face-to-face consultation, either the patient then leaves the room and the neurologist talks to the doctor or nurse, or the consultation is terminated; this is a lot easier to do over a videolink than with face-to-face consultation, as it involves simply pressing a button!

Discussion with doctors

For inpatients, where a doctor is with the patient, it is important to discuss the diagnosis and management with them to ensure that there are no misunderstandings. The doctor then writes a summary of this discussion in the hospital case notes. This part of the procedure has considerable educational value for doctors in training, who may seldom have witnessed a properly conducted neurological assessment, and it is important that there is an opportunity for the presenting doctor to ask questions or seek clarification.

After the call is closed

Once reality returns and the television doctor is no longer present, the patient may remember other facts, ask further questions or make important comments that did not come out during the consultation. This is a feature of telemedicine not usually found in face-to-face consultations. The nurse or doctor who will have witnessed the consultation will usually be able to deal with these, but the neurologist may need to be consulted either by reconnecting the call or by telephoning them. Often, the sentiment is one of relief: 'I'm glad they said I didn't have motor neurone disease. My best friend's father has just died of that.'

Recording the consultation

It is important that a record of the consultation with the imprimatur of the neurologist appears in the patient's case notes. For outpatients, we use a standard letter dictated by the neurologist and transferred to the secretary at the referring hospital. For inpatients, we use a standard form dictated by the neurologist and typed by the teleneurology coordinator and then faxed or emailed to the referring hospital (Fig. 12.9). We also record details of each inpatient consultation on a spreadsheet. It is important that the activity is recorded on the hospital system. We record these either as new outpatient attendances or as inpatient consultations on the patient-administration system of the referring hospital.

Intercontinental Teleneurology Consultation to the COH, Brisbane

Teleneurology number	IC 007
Patient's name	
Unit no.	
DOB	3/12/87
Date of admission	
Date of consultation	

History

Flu 3/52 ago with pains, recovered but mother said v. pale today, fainted at church – felt heart racing, cold and shivered, out for < 1 min sore back and both legs after and diff standing, now only sore R leg. Faint once before.

Examination

SLR 40°R, 85°L. Pain on LS ext and R side fl. No neurological signs

Diagnosis

faint, sciatica

Investigations

Lumbar spine X-ray

Treatment

Physio, encouragement

Disposal

Home am, no neuro review

Seen By

Vp/jm

Fig. 12.9. Record of consultation (anonymized) sent to the referring hospital.

Conclusion

In teleneurology, as in other walks of life, attention to detail pays dividends. It is possible to perform real-time videoconferencing without many of the above structures, but failure is more likely and the process will not flow as smoothly. The five essential principles are:

 it must be as easy as possible for the presenting doctor/nurse

- ▶ the rooms must be well-lit and have good acoustics
- ▶ adequate bandwidth must be used
- ▶ a videoconferencing expert must be available continuously by telephone in case things go wrong
- ▶ the process needs to be timetabled at both ends.

The challenge of real-time teleneurology for the neurologist is that it requires a subtle but significant change in how neurology is practised. For example, watching someone else perform a neurological examination can be difficult until you realize that if you cannot see a sign demonstrated in this way, then it probably is not there. Making these changes is worth it for the neurologist because of the improvements in service that real-time teleneurology can offer patients.

Further information

Tachakra S, Sivakumar A, Hayes J, Dawood M. A protocol for telemedical consultation. *Journal of Telemedicine and Telecare* 1997; **3**: 163–168.

References

1   Wootton R. Telemedicine: a cautious welcome. *British Medical Journal* 1996; **313**: 1375–1377.
2   Falconer J. Telemedicine systems and telecommunications. In *Introduction to Telemedicine*. Wootton R, Craig J, eds. London: Royal Society of Medicine Press, 1999; pp 17–36.
3   Major J. Telemedicine room design. *Journal of Telemedicine and Telecare* 2005; **11**: 10–14.
4   Patterson V. Teleneurology in Northern Ireland: a success. *Journal of Telemedicine and Telecare* 2002; **8** (suppl. 3): 46–47.

Websites for Neurologists

Rustam Al-Shahi

The World Wide Web: the teleneurologist's second home

Not even the most sceptical neurologist can deny the current and future importance of the World Wide Web to their practice: patients use it before seeing doctors[1] and doctors use it after seeing patients.[2] As the web proliferates, and access to it increases, at least in the industrialized world, any 'neurosceptics' will find the medium inescapable.

Meanwhile, enlightened web-friendly neurologists, amongst whom all teleneurologists must surely be included, need to rely on – and keep up to date with – the best of the web. Rather than attempt a comprehensive summary, which is probably impossible, I have distilled the adult/child neurology and clinical neurophysiology resources down to a manageable list of high-quality websites (Table 13.1). My recommendations are based on a series of review articles that appeared in the *Journal of Neurology, Neurosurgery and Psychiatry* (*JNNP*) in the period 2002–03 that covered Internet concepts and websites for medicine in general,[3] neurosurgery and neuropathology,[4] psychiatry and neuropsychiatry,[5] and adult/child neurology and clinical neurophysiology.[6] I also conducted a PubMed search up to 1 January 2005 using the medical subject heading (MeSH) term 'Internet' combined with the MeSH term 'neurology', and reviewed the *Journal of the American Medical Informatics Association* and other web sources.

Although the web is a truly global medium, the sites I have included (especially the professional organizations listed in Table 13.3) in this chapter are slightly biased by my country of residence. Thus, some websites may have been omitted because there is a UK equivalent of similar quality. For websites mentioned in the text but not listed in the tables, uniform resource locators (URLs) are provided in the text.

Before you start: optimize your browser

Browsers are software applications that create a user-friendly window for many of the Internet services. Browser technology is developing continuously. Although the two main browsers are Microsoft Internet Explorer (www.microsoft.com/windows/ie/) and Netscape Navigator (http://home.netscape.com), there are many others available for the web aficionado (see www.browsers.com). You should ensure that you use the latest version of your browser. The current browser series for use with recent operating systems is 6.*x* (the decimal after the series number is the version number, denoting new features and fixed program bugs).

Table 13.1. Useful websites for neurologists (accessed 7 January 2005)

Site name	URL	Site description
Medical portals		
National electronic Library for Health (NeLH)	www.nelh.nhs.uk	Partnership with NHS Libraries to develop a digital library for NHS staff, patients and the public
TRIP database	www.tripdatabase.com	Free searchable database of over 55 sources of high-quality evidence-based information and online journals
Scottish Intercollegiate Guidelines Network	www.sign.ac.uk	Public resource for evidence-based clinical practice guidelines from the UK
National Guideline Clearing House	www.guideline.gov	Public resource for evidence-based clinical practice guidelines from the USA
Netting the Evidence	www.shef.ac.uk/scharr/ir/netting/	Comprehensive resource for evidence-based practice
American Academy of Neurology practice guidelines	www.aan.com/professionals/ practice/guidelines.cfm	North American evidence-based aids to clinical decision-making
Neurosciences on the Internet	www.neuroguide.com	Comprehensive directory of Internet neuroscience resources
BIOME	http://biome.ac.uk	Searchable catalogue of quality Internet health and biomedical resources, and incorporating Organising Medical Networked Information
Doctors.net	www.doctors.net.uk	Free news, discussion, literature, jobs and email service for UK doctors
Medical conferences	www.medicalconferences.com	Interactive free compendium of worldwide medical conferences
General journals		
PubMed	www.ncbi.nlm.nih.gov/entrez	Searchable version of MEDLINE with links to online journals, and integrated with other protein, nucleotide and genome databases
PubMed Central	http://pubmedcentral.nih.gov	Digital archive of life sciences journal literature
Free Medical Journals	www.freemedicaljournals.com	Portal dedicated to indexing and promoting free access to medical journals on the web
Public Library of Science	www.plos.org	Non-profit-making organization of scientists and physicians committed to making the world's scientific and medical literature a freely available public resource, see Fig. 13.1
Zetoc	http://zetoc.mimas.ac.uk	The British Library's email service for all of its journals' latest tables of contents
BioMed Central	www.biomedcentral.com	Independent publishing house committed to providing immediate free access to peer-reviewed biomedical research
Textbooks		
FreeBooks4Doctors	www.freebooks4doctors.com	Portal dedicated to free access to medical books on the web
eMedicine	www.emedicine.com	Free web-only textbook of medicine, with sponsorship by the pharmaceutical industry

Table 13.1. – continued

Site name	URL	Site description
eMedicine Neurology	www.emedicine.com/neuro	Neurology section of eMedicine
Neuromuscular Diseases textbook	www.neuro.wustl. edu/neuromuscular	Free multi-authored textbook dedicated to neuromuscular diseases
MedLink eurology	www.medlink.com	Subscription-only neurology textbook
Research resources		
Cochrane Library	www.thecochranelibrary.com	Synthesis of reliable evidence about the effects of healthcare
Cochrane Neurological Network	www.cochraneneuronet.org	Functions as a link between neurologists and the Cochrane Collaboration
Current Controlled Trials	www.controlled-trials.com	Promotes the availability and exchange of information about ongoing randomized controlled trials in all areas of healthcare
PubCrawler	http://pubcrawler.gen.tcd.ie	Free alerting service that scans daily updates to the PubMed and GenBank databases
Paediatric neurology		
Child-Neuro.Org.UK	www.child-neuro.org.uk	Gateway to news, education, information and discussion about child neurology
Child Neurology	www.waisman.wisc.edu/ child-neuro/	Portal for paediatric neurology resources
Online Mendelian Inheritance in Man	www.ncbi.nlm.nih.gov/omim/	Catalogue of genes and genetic disorders
Clinical neurophysiology		
Clinical Neurophysiology	www.clinicalneurophysiology. org.uk	British portal for clinical neurophysiology web resources
TeleEMG.com	www.teleemg.com	Useful information for clinical neurophysiologists, with an online store and doctor/patient discussion groups
News and discussion		
Neurologist discussion list	www.neurolist.com/site	Email discussion list for neurologists
NeurologyLinx	www.neurologylinx.com	Web-based and emailed daily news about general neurology and subspecialties

Table 13.2 contains a list of recommended ways of optimizing your browser. Security deserves a special mention. The reference standard for web security is the Secure Sockets Layer (SSL) protocol and the Secure Hypertext Transport Protocol (SHTTP). A URL that begins with https:// indicates a secure server, which is denoted by a closed padlock symbol on the status bar of your browser. It is your responsibility, however, to ensure that SSL is activated under Tools/Internet Options/Content in your browser: the server checks only that you enter the SSL port, not whether your browser is actually using SSL.

Table 13.2. Enhance your use of a browser

Maintain software:
Use the latest version of a browser, eg Microsoft Internet Explorer (IE) (determine which version you are using by looking under Help/About Internet Explorer)
Update your browser with the latest security patches (http://windowsupdate.microsoft.com/)
Use the latest versions of free software to view multimedia content:
    Paint Shop Pro (www.jasc.com)
    Adobe Acrobat Reader (www.adobe.com/prodindex/acrobat)
    Shockwave (www.macromedia.com/shockwave/)
    QuickTime (www.quicktime.com)
    RealPlayer (www.real.com)
Install virus protection software and keep it up-to-date (www.symantec.com, www.mcafee.com, www.zonelabs.com)

Shorten the time you spend online:
Download only text and omit multimedia content if the bandwidth of your connection is low*
If you pay for the time you are connected to an Internet service provider (ISP), then download pages as you browse in separate windows (hold down the Shift key while you click on links) and read them later when you are offline

Minimize memory use:
Set your History folder to store web pages only for as long as you will need them*
Optimize the size of your cache/Temporary Internet Files folder*

Customize your browser:
Set your browser's home page to a blank page (about:blank) or the website that you use the most*
Organize your Favorites/Bookmarks into folders
Set your preferred font type* and size (under View/Text Size)
Maximize the viewable area in your browser by removing the explorer bar and customizing toolbars to show only the functions you use (as small icons)*
Use the appropriate default programs for sending email etc. from your browser*

Take shortcuts:
When typing uniform resource locators (URLs), omit http:// as your browser will automatically append it
Use copy and paste functions to transfer URLs between documents and browser
Right-click with your mouse to save images, sounds or videos from a website to your hard drive
If a website cannot be found with the URL you have entered, try shortening it from the right-hand end towards the domain name, or use a search engine

---

*Change these by going to Tools/Internet Options in your browser.

Other browser security measures to be taken include using the current version of your browser (which will be compatible with the latest security software and have known security risks protected), setting the level of security to medium or high (in Tools/Internet Options), disabling AutoComplete functions for forms (to stop your browser storing your passwords), and disabling embedded client-side programming languages (such as Java), which would otherwise expose your browser to threats from applets that could exploit the data on your computer.

Cookies are small files placed on your computer by a website host server (www.cookiecentral.com). Because some Internet Protocol (IP) addresses are not static but are allocated dynamically (ie when you dial in to an Internet service provider (ISP), they are allocated from its limited pool of IP addresses), cookies were developed to enable their website of origin to recognize a specific returning user. By aiding recognition, cookies speed up logging into password-protected zones and allow personalization of web content; they also help website developers to assess their site's traffic and monitor viewing habits. Clearly, using cookies is unwise on shared computers, but it will be a matter of personal preference as to whether you accept them and whether you enable the cookie-alerting mechanism in your browser. The only cost of greater security, of course, is that you will be unable to benefit from the enhancements offered by cookies and Java applets.

Although extra windows that 'pop up' when you visit websites are sometimes helpful (eg seeing larger versions of images), they are usually unwanted. Unfortunately, some pop-up windows can contain inappropriate content or can be a way for you to accidentally download dangerous software (called spyware or adware) on to your computer. With Windows XP Service Pack 2 (SP2), Internet Explorer allows you to block pop-up windows and customize those that you wish to appear.

World Wide Web resources

Search engines, subject directories and search agents

The websites that help you find your way around the web are freely accessible. They may be *search engines* (eg www.google.com), which scour the web itself for sites of relevance, *directories* of sites compiled and reviewed by the authors of the directory (eg http://dmoz.org), *hybrids* of the two (eg www.altavista.com) or *search agents* (eg www.copernic.com).

Search engines are valuable for their sensitivity, whereas directories have a higher specificity[7]. Up-to-date information on the relative merits of the different engines is available from a site called Search Engine Watch (www.searchenginewatch.com). Because of the way it compiles its index, Google is by far and away the largest of the engines at present. For example, in 0.12 seconds, the Google search engine retrieves over 6.9 million websites relating to the search term 'neurology' from its computer-generated index of web content. But, however fast and sensitive search engines are, they are best searched with more specific criteria[3,7]. For the hurried neurologist, a search engine will often provide something of relevance, but it may not be of the best quality.

Subject directories – also called gateways and portals – are usually indexed in a hierarchical file structure and are rated by the people who compile them. Thus, information local to the UK, for example, is best found on the regional version of the directory (eg http://uk.yahoo.com rather than www.yahoo.com). Google's directory yields a mere 7350 websites using the same search criterion as I used above, and the websites are ranked by their perceived order of relevance. Although directories have a health category, the highest-quality medical information is to be found on specialist portals (see below).

Crucial to finding the website closest to your requirements is to use search terms that are most specific to your needs and yet are sensitive enough not to miss anything useful. It is most important to read the 'About' section of the search engine or directory that you choose to use. Engines can search for particular types of file (eg web pages, sound files, graphics), in certain languages, and use suggested keywords and employ Boolean commands (eg to incorporate multiple terms or to exclude other terms). Undoubtedly the most powerful method of finding the information you want is to use a search agent, such as Copernic, which automatically searches multiple search engines and directories with your search terms, removes duplicates, and compiles and ranks the results.

Many of the search tools offer a free downloadable toolbar for your web browser, which allows direct entry of a search term, saving a visit to the website of the search engine. For example, http://toolbar.google.com provides a toolbar with all of Google's search capabilities, as well as a pop-up blocker, online form auto completion with one click, personalized search engine options, and highlighting of your search term(s) on the page you visit.

General medical portals

The accessibility, format and functionality of the web enable medical portals to come into their own in providing indexed comprehensive databases of high-quality information, and allow journals and even textbooks to be reproduced online.[8,9] However, there is a profusion of medical portals offering these collated resources to doctors and patients, or both (generally from North America with URLs beginning www.med. or www.MD.), and sometimes requiring a subscription. Some portals, such as doctors.net.uk, go even further to try and foster an online community by offering other services, such as discussion forums, a searchable database of colleagues, a classified section, server space for document storage and e-commerce.

The TRIP database is perhaps the most user-friendly, evidence-based resource for neurologists. It is designed to bring together all the evidence-based healthcare resources available on the Internet, and it provides a free search of the main evidence-based resources, peer-reviewed journals, guidelines and e-textbooks on the web. It has a dedicated neurology 'clinical area', which issues monthly updates that can be received by email.

The TRIP database includes coverage of the Cochrane Library, which has review groups dedicated to dementia and cognitive impairment, epilepsy, movement disorders, multiple sclerosis, neuromuscular disorders and stroke. Although the Cochrane Library operates on a subscription basis, free access is provided to low-income countries, and many countries have arranged national provisions (http://www3.interscience.wiley.com/cgi-bin/mrwhome/106568753/DoYouAlreadyHaveAccess.html). For example, in the UK the full text of the library can be accessed via the National electronic Library for Health (NeLH), which aims to deliver high-quality information to improve patient care in the National Health Service (NHS).[10] The NeLH is a gateway for staff in the NHS to access a variety of resources, primarily concerning evidence-based medicine. Whereas only the abstracts of reviews in the Cochrane Library are available to anyone on the web (www.thecochranelibrary.com), the NeLH provides the entire contents of the Cochrane Library. Similarly, access to the entire contents of *Clinical Evidence* (www.clinicalevidence.com) and evidence-based on call (www.eboncall.org) are available via the NeLH. There are links to PubMed and a comprehensive database of guidelines from sources such as the Scottish Intercollegiate Guidelines Network (SIGN), the National Institute of Clinical Excellence (NICE) (www.nice.org.uk) and the US-based National Guideline Clearing House.

Neurology portals

Neurology portals are distinguished from each other by various attributes, including the comprehensiveness of their selection of websites, any bias in their compilation (in language, country of origin, funding or disease category), the sophistication of software for searching the directory, and their presentation. Because readers are likely to use at most a handful of portals to direct their further browsing, I have been rather selective. Although the dot.com world is now relatively impoverished, forcing medical website developers to resort to advertising, I have tried to avoid recommending sponsored sites because they are likely to be biased in their content.

Neurology portals can be divided into two types:

Evidence-based neurology portals
The Cochrane Neurological Network functions as a link between neurologists and the Cochrane Collaboration. Guidelines for the practice of clinical neurology are not as yet united on one website, presumably because they tend to vary by region. The American Academy of Neurology (AAN) practice guidelines, which are kept updated, are freely available as portable document format (PDF) files on the AAN website.

General neurology portals
Without doubt, the single most useful directory for neurologists is Neurosciences on the Internet. This website was established in 1994, and its coverage of clinical neuroscience is strong, including lists of other portals, disease-related websites, patients' organizations, mailing lists and discussion groups, educational resources and useful software; it has a slight North American bias. Other directories simply do not compare, so I suggest it should be the starting point for a survey of web resources in any particular area of neurology. Whilst many websites devoted to particular categories of neurological disorder are worthy of mention (eg www.wemove.org dedicated to worldwide education and awareness for movement disorders), the majority are indexed by Neurosciences on the Internet. Professional organizations' websites (Table 13.3) often provide good guidance on websites appropriate to their region.

Journals

Internet idealists see the web as the most revolutionary development in publishing since the printing press. Online repositories for articles, such as BioMed Central and PubMed Central, have embraced the idea of free access for all to the medical

Table 13.3. Professional organizations (incomplete list) (accessed 7 January 2005)

Site name	URL	Site description
Association of British Neurologists	www.theabn.org	Professional association for British neurologists
American Neurological Association	www.aneuroa.org	Professional association of North American neurologists
American Academy of Neurology	www.aan.com	Resources for professional and practice development for neurologists
World Federation of Neurology	www.wfneurology.org	Promotes worldwide practice, education and research in neurology, in association with the WHO
European Neurological Society	www.ensinfo.com	Promotes neurology – especially education and research – in Europe
European Federation of Neurological Societies	www.efns.org	Promotes neurology – especially education and research – in Europe
British Paediatric Neurology Association	www.bpna.org.uk	Professional association for British paediatric neurologists
International Child Neurology Association	www.child-neuro.net/	Professional association for paediatric neurologists worldwide
Child Neurology Society	www.childneurologysociety.org	Professional association for North American paediatric neurologists
British Society for Clinical Neurophysiology	www.bscn.org.uk	Professional association to promote and assist the science and practice of clinical neurophysiology
American Clinical Neurophysiology Society	www.acns.org	Professional association for clinical neurophysiologists
American Academy of Clinical Neurophysiology	www.aacnonline.com	Dedicated to communication amongst clinical and basic neurophysiologists
American Association of Neuromuscular and Electrodiagnostic Medicine	www.aanem.org	Professional association for clinical neurophysiologists, affiliated to the AMA
International Federation of Clinical Neurophysiology	www.ifcn.info	Promotes education and research in clinical neurophysiology

AMA, American Medical Association; WHO, World Health Organization.

literature,[11] known as open-access publishing.[12] PubMed Central provides free access to some print journals already offering their entire contents online (eg www.bmj.com) in addition to the purely electronic journals in BioMed Central (eg *BMC Neurology*: www.biomedcentral.com/bmcneurol) and the recent Public Library of Science (Fig. 13.1). Authors of articles in these reservoirs of knowledge benefit from being indexed in PubMed, from being published the moment they are accepted, and from not having to transfer copyright to the publisher. Free Medical Journals provides a comprehensive list of medical journals that are either free at the point of publication or after a delay, and the Directory of Open Access Journals (www.doaj.org) indexes free, full-text, quality-controlled scientific and scholarly journals in all subjects and languages.

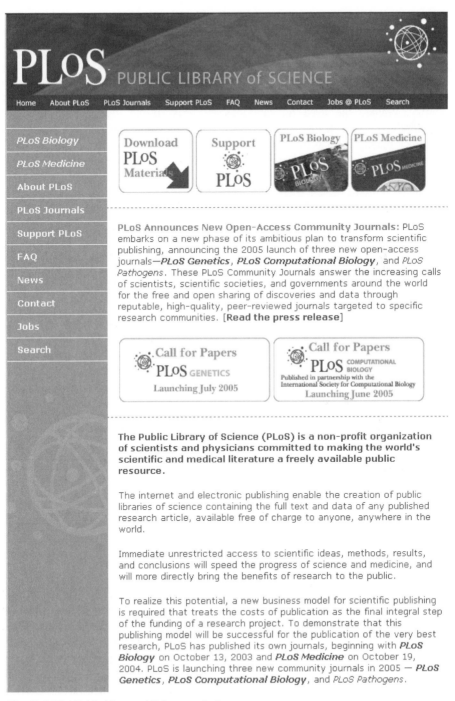

Fig. 13.1. The Public Library of Science website.

There are several other advantages of online publication, such as the speedy dissemination of preprints or 'netprints' (research before, during or after review by other agencies), web-based supplements to print articles (which are likely to improve the quality of reporting),[13] and preprint servers (which might help to prevent publication bias).[14] Hypertext links between reference lists from an article in one online journal and the original article in another, and from portals direct to the online journal, obviate the need for laborious journeys to the library. Online article submission enables faster peer review. Article citations can be downloaded to reference-management software or downloaded as PDF files for printing in a format indistinguishable from the paper version of the article. Moreover, free full-text access can be delivered to resource-poor countries.

Finally, journals' emailed tables of contents (eTOCs) and automatic alerts about articles on particular topics or by particular authors can result in a more time-effective way of keeping up to date. Signing up for an eTOC is usually done through an online journal's website, a subscription to the journal usually is not required, and removing oneself from the list is as easy as signing up. An excellent eTOC service offered for any journal received by the British Library (regardless of whether the journal provides an eTOC of its own) is available from Zetoc, which can be accessed freely via the NeLH.

Despite the advantages, some view online journals as a threat to the 'integrity of the scholarly record of science',[15] and resent the loss of the aesthetic appeal of a paper journal. Publishing houses fear a greater burden for peer review with easier article submission, loss of copyright, and lower revenue from print subscriptions, which are only slightly offset by online subscriptions and pay-per-article fees, themselves jeopardized by unlegislated peer-to-peer information-sharing technology. The main fear is that open-access journals will not be able to maintain the conventional standard of peer review.

Almost every neurology journal has a website that can provide the full text of recent issues. Sometimes, only abstracts or tables of contents are available. Table 13.4 lists a small selection of clinical neurology journals, ranked by their impact factor; a more complete list is available from Neurosciences on the Internet and from PubMed's journal database. Most online journals are reproductions of their print counterparts. However, some peer-reviewed journals exist only in electronic format, *BMC Neurology* being the main example. One of the many advantages of the electronic format is the cross-referencing of bibliographies using citation-linking.

Sadly, the ideal of open-access publishing has not yet been realized in neurology, and full-text access mostly requires a paid subscription. Although Free Medical Journals lists 37 neurology journals, the degree of access varies from complete availability to only articles published more than two years ago. Some journals offer the alternative of purchasing individual articles. Without a subscription, many offer free access to selected articles from each issue, and most provide article abstracts and eTOC services. If eTOCs are not available from the journal itself, then various alerting services exist to provide a comprehensive eTOC,[3] whilst news services (see below) provide edited synopses.

Table 13.4. Popular clinical neurology journal* websites (accessed 7 January 2005)

Journal	URL	Free full text?	eTOC?
Annals of Neurology	www.interscience.wiley.com/jpages/0364-5134	No	Yes
Brain	http://brain.oupjournals.org	Articles > 2 years old	Yes
Journal of Neuropathology and Experimental Neurology	http://neur.allenpress.com/neuronline/?request=index-html	No	Yes
Stroke	http://intl-stroke.ahajournals.org	Articles > 1 year old	Yes
Neurology	http://intl.neurology.org	No	Yes
Archives of Neurology	http://archneur.ama-assn.org	No	Yes
Current Opinion in Neurology	www.co-neurology.com	No	Yes
Cephalalgia	www.blackwellpublishing.com/journals/cha	No	Yes
Epilepsia	www.epilepsia.com	No	Yes
Journal of Neurology, Neurosurgery and Psychiatry	www.jnnp.com	Articles > 1 year old	Yes
Practical Neurology	www.blackwell-science.com/pnr	No	Yes

*Journals selected are based partly on their impact factors provided by the Institute for Scientific Information.
eTOC, emailed table of contents.

e-Textbooks

General medical e-textbooks that are available electronically can be found via FreeBooks4Doctors, which is a portal dedicated to indexing textbooks that are freely available on the web, whether purely electronic or not. At the forefront, eMedicine is a comprehensive, entirely web-based e-textbook and portal, requiring only registration and no paid subscription. Despite the appearance of sponsors and advertising on this website, authors are independent of the pharmaceutical industry. UpToDate (www.uptodate.com) is an independent e-textbook, but it requires a subscription. The majority of printed medical textbooks with an online version require a subscription, such as Harrison's Online (www.harrisonsonline.com), which is an expanded, continually updated, cross-referenced version of the sixteenth edition of *Harrison's Principles of Internal Medicine*. Other textbooks, such as the *Oxford Textbook of Medicine*, are only available for purchase as a CD-ROM, although Doctors.net.uk does provide free full-text access to this textbook for its members.

There are two web-based textbooks dedicated to general neurology. eMedicine Neurology is a North American multi-authored work that is freely accessible with registration; it is searchable, well designed and comprehensive. MedLink Neurology is a subscription-only North American electronic textbook (available on the web and as a CD-ROM updated quarterly), which also includes neurosurgery topics, videos and a discussion board, but it costs at least US$299 per year. The Neuromuscular Diseases textbook is an unrivalled speciality resource that provides open-access, up-to-date, comprehensive, intuitively indexed medical and patient information.

Many of the resources cited above offer text and picture content suitable for creating lectures. Additional teaching resources include www.neuroexam.com, which illustrates the various stages of the neurological examination with streaming video, and the Eye Simulator (http://cim.ucdavis.edu/EyeRelease), which accurately simulates eye movements and pupillary responses in both health and disease. Neurologists wishing to test their knowledge on a regular basis can attempt to diagnose the Baylor College of Medicine case of the month, using the history and examination provided with an interactive battery of tests, and then return to the website the following month for the denouement (www.bcm.tmc.edu/neurol/case.html).

Research

Although medical portals compile evidence-based resources and journals for use in clinical practice and research, a valuable tool for researchers to keep up to date is PubCrawler – a free alerting service that scans daily updates to PubMed and GenBank databases ('It goes to the library. You go to the pub' is its stated modus operandi). National and international repositories of research activity are of particular value to researchers. Registries of ongoing and completed studies are important to prevent unnecessary duplication and publication bias and can provide paradigms for other areas where research is needed. For example, the National Research Register (www.update-software.com/National) compiles data about research activity in the UK, whilst Current Controlled Trials and Centerwatch (www.centerwatch.com) collate information about randomized controlled trials in particular.

News and discussion

Mailing lists, newsgroups, bulletin boards, web forums and chat rooms offer online communities in which peers can exchange news, opinions and comment. Mailing lists usually are administered by a host institution and use software such as Listserv (www.lsoft.com) to circulate emailed contributions to a discussion on a particular topic. Joining a list is initiated simply by sending an email to the administrative address (the membership of some lists is vetted); anonymity is maintained unless you wish to contribute, and content is usually moderated. A good starting point would be the 'Medicine and Health' category at www.jiscmail.ac.uk. Newsgroups (such as misc.health and sci.med, available via http://groups.google.com), bulletin boards and web forums offer a similar, but web-based, means of communication that does not clog up your email inbox.

NeurologyLinx is a website dedicated to providing news about both general and specialized neurology. Although the website is sponsored, its advertisers do not influence content. News is updated daily on the website and in email bulletins, which comprise mostly information from journals and conferences.

Newsgroups offer an often unrestricted, interactive, web-based means of exchanging news and (mostly) views.[3] At the time of writing, there were about 47 000 newsgroups. Their index – Google Groups – did not list a dedicated neurology group, although at first glance bionet.neuroscience appeared to qualify. However, bionet.neuroscience contained about 34 000 discussion threads, most of which were unscientific. There are newsgroups dedicated to particular diseases (eg sci.med.diseases.als, sci.med.diseases.alzheimer, sci.med.diseases.lyme, sci.med.diseases.mult-sclerosis), although neurologists are unlikely to find these of use in their speciality. Some patients may benefit from discussions with others in the alt.support.disorders.neurological newsgroup.

Email discussion lists provide a more secure forum for neurologists to discuss professional issues by email. One of the longest established lists of this nature is the Neurologist Discussion List, vetted by a neurologist at the Medical College of Georgia.[16] Members admitted to this list can control the frequency and content of email messages that update them about ongoing discussions. Although posts to this list may often discuss issues such as computer software, caution has been urged in the discussion of patient management because the legal status of advice proffered or heeded is unclear.[17] Neurosciences on the Internet (www.neuroguide.com/neurolist.html) has compiled the contact details of many other email discussion lists (ranging from special interests in neurology, to paediatric neurology and clinical neurophysiology).

Patients

Because Internet access and usage are rising dramatically, and health is one of the main categories of information sought, the provision of high-quality patient information is essential. Although some have doubted the importance of this phenomenon,[18] a recent survey found that one-quarter of patients with home access to the Internet used medical websites before consultation at a neurology clinic, and this information was inappropriate in 60% of cases.[1] Because misinformation may be harmful due to incorrect self-diagnosis, inappropriate treatment discontinuation or self-medication, and the potential of the Internet to encourage suicide, organizations exist to monitor health fraud on the web (www.quackwatch.com).

The Health on the Net Foundation (www.hon.ch) is a not-for-profit organization established to guide patients and medical practitioners to useful and reliable online health and medical information, guided by their established code of conduct. Possibly the best websites for providing patients with information about the whole range of medical conditions are Patient UK, Healthsites and MedicDirect in the UK and www.healthfinder.gov in the USA.

Portals supplying patient information of uniformly high quality about the whole breadth of neurological diseases are hard to find (Table 13.5), but the US National Institute of Neurologic Disorders and Stroke (NINDS) comes close. The National Organization for Rare Disorders (NORD) is a useful supplement to the NINDS website, especially for physicians based in the USA. MEDLINEplus (www.nlm.nih.gov/medlineplus/neurologicdiseasesgeneral.html) provides comprehensive patient information (mostly from the NINDS website), with further links to news, diagrams, research, organizations and medical dictionaries. In the UK, the Neurological Alliance has collated links to the major patient support organizations, one of which is the Brain and Spine Foundation, which publishes a growing number of well-written and freely downloadable information leaflets.

Patients' further needs for communication and discussion can be fulfilled in disease-specific online support groups via some of these websites. Where this is lacking, many

Table 13.5. Useful websites for patients (accessed 7 January 2005)

Site name	URL	Site description
Information		
Patient UK	www.patient.co.uk	Directory of UK health- and disease-related websites for patients
Healthsites	www.healthsites.co.uk	Portal for health-related information, with sections for patients and doctors
medicdirect	www.medicdirect.co.uk	Portal for health-related information for both patients and doctors
QuackWatch	www.quackwatch.com	Surveillance of bogus health websites
National Institute of Neurologic Disorders and Stroke	www.ninds.nih.gov	USA-based funding and information resource
National Organization for Rare Disorders	www.rarediseases.org	US federation of voluntary health organizations dedicated to rare disorders
Neurological Alliance	http://neural.org.uk	UK alliance of charities dedicated to neurological diseases
Brain and Spine Foundation	www.brainandspine.org.uk	Foundation to develop research, education and information about neurological disorders
News and discussion		
BrainTalk Communities	www.braintalk.org	Online discussion forums for patients with neurological illnesses
Massachusetts General Hospital neurology chat rooms	www.BrainChat.org	Online discussion forums for patients with neurological illnesses

patients – particularly those in the USA – join the web-based BrainTalk communities or the Massachusetts General Hospital neurology chat rooms to interact with over 50 000 others about general and specific neurological conditions.

Child neurology

The best resource for child neurology is Child-Neuro.Org.UK, which, despite its emphasis, is an up-to-date source of links, news, discussion and practice resources for paediatric neurologists worldwide. The Child Neurology website had been the leading paediatric neurology portal for some time.[19] It also runs the Child-Neuro email discussion list (www.waisman.wisc.edu/archives/child-neuro.html). Paediatric neurologists will also find the Neuromuscular Disease Center and Online Mendelian Inheritance in Man (OMIM) particularly valuable resources for up-to-date information about neuromuscular and genetic diseases, respectively.

Tables of contents and email alerts are available – sometimes requiring registration – for the main journals, *Developmental Medicine and Child Neurology* (www.journals.cambridge.org/journal_DevelopmentalMedicineandChildNeurology), *Neuropediatrics* (www.thieme.de/neuropediatrics) and *Journal of Child Neurology* (www.bcdecker.com/aiDetails.aspx?aiiID=6), but free access is not provided to the full text of the online journals.

Clinical neurophysiology

There are three main portals for clinical neurophysiologists, each with its own merits. TeleEMG.com provides a wealth of resources [an online electromyography (EMG) manual, educational aids, a practical guide for electromyographers, the TeleEMG calculator for comparing sensory and motor conduction velocities with controls, and discussion groups].[20] However, TeleEMG.com is a for-profit website that sells some of these products as well as the EMG assistant diagnostic program (www.emgassistant.com). Clinical Neurophysiology is a very well designed website with many up-to-date informative links, but some sections remain under development. Less impressive is Clinical Neurophysiology on the Internet (www.neurophys.com).

Both tables of contents and email alerts are available for the two main journals dedicated to clinical neurophysiology, *Journal of Clinical Neurophysiology* (www.clinicalneurophys.com) and *Clinical Neurophysiology* (www.sciencedirect.com/science/journal/13882457), but neither allows free access to the full text of the online journal.

Conclusion

There is no reason to be daunted by the quantity of information about neurology on the web. Large quantities of high-quality information are provided by a small selection of portals, and it seems intuitive that better access to them should improve the standard of healthcare, although this remains unproven in a formal sense. Whilst the Internet has not yet usurped neurologists' diagnostic skills, online diagnostic tools are already available as adjuncts to neurologists' knowledge (http://simulconsult.com).

The websites listed in this chapter, and others recommended in the *JNNP* Internet review series,[3–6] can be downloaded easily from www.jnnp.com and incorporated into your web browser as a Bookmark/Favorite file. Keeping abreast of the further progress of neurological knowledge merely requires neurologists to embrace the concept of being updated by email and to keep an eye on their favourite websites.

Further information

The *JNNP* provides a monthly review of neurological websites: http://jnnp.bmjjournals.com/cgi/collection/internet. Accessed 23 January 2005.

References

1 Larner AJ. Use of internet medical websites and NHS direct by neurology outpatients before consultation. *International Journal of Clinical Practice* 2002; **56**: 219–221.

2 Westbrook JI, Gosling AS, Coiera E. Do clinicians use online evidence to support patient care? A study of 55,000 clinicians. *Journal of the American Medical Informatics Association* 2004; **11**: 113–120.

3   Al-Shahi R, Sadler M, Rees G, Bateman D. The internet. *Journal of Neurology, Neurosurgery and Psychiatry* 2002; **73**: 619–628.

4   Thomson S, Phillips N. Internet resources for neurosurgeons and neuropathologists. *Journal of Neurology, Neurosurgery and Psychiatry* 2003; **74**: 154–157.

5   Stone J, Sharpe M. Internet resources for psychiatry and neuropsychiatry. *Journal of Neurology, Neurosurgery and Psychiatry* 2003; **74**: 10–12.

6   Al-Shahi R, Sandercock PA. Internet resources for neurologists. *Journal of Neurology, Neurosurgery and Psychiatry* 2003; **74**: 699-703.

7   Al-Shahi R. Search engines. *Practical Neurology* 2001; **1**: 60–61.

8   Hunt DL, Jaeschke R, McKibbon KA. Users' guides to the medical literature: XXI. Using electronic health information resources in evidence-based practice. Evidence-Based Medicine Working Group. *Journal of the American Medical Association* 2000; **283**: 1875–1879.

9   Jadad AR, Haynes RB, Hunt D, Browman GP. The Internet and evidence-based decision-making: a needed synergy for efficient knowledge management in health care. *Canadian Medical Association Journal* 2000; **162**: 362–365.

10   Muir Gray JA, de Lusignan S. National electronic Library for Health (NeLH). *British Medical Journal* 1999; **319**: 1476–1479.

11   Delamothe T, Smith R. PubMed Central: creating an Aladdin's cave of ideas. *British Medical Journal* 2001; **322**: 1–2.

12   Delamothe T, Smith R. Open access publishing takes off. *British Medical Journal* 2004; **328**: 1–3.

13   Chalmers I, Altman DG. How can medical journals help prevent poor medical research? Some opportunities presented by electronic publishing. *Lancet* 1999; **353**: 490–493.

14   Song F, Eastwood A, Gilbody S, Duley L. The role of electronic journals in reducing publication bias. *Medical Informatics and the Internet in Medicine* 1999; **24**: 223–229.

15   Lindberg DA, Humphreys BL. Medicine and health on the Internet: the good, the bad, and the ugly. *Journal of the American Medical Association* 1998; **280**: 1303–1304.

16   Rivner MH. Neuro@neurolist.mcg.edu: an e-mail discussion list for neurologists. *Neurology* 1999; **52**: 1891–1893.

17   Beresford HR, Brooke MH. The Webster's dictionary: neurologists on the Internet. *Neurology* 1999; **52**: 1730–1731.

18   Jadad AR, Sigouin C, Cocking L *et al.* Internet use among physicians, nurses, and their patients. *Journal of the American Medical Association* 2001; **286**: 1451–1452.

19   Leber S, Mack K. The Internet and clinical practice of child neurology. *Current Opinion in Neurology* 2000; **13**: 147–153.

20   Jabre JF, Stalberg EV, Bassi R. TeleMedicine and Internet EMG. *Supplements to Clinical Neurophysiology* 2000; **53**: 163–167.

▶14

Neurology Tele-education

John McConville

Introduction

Sir William Osler famously said: 'To study the phenomenon of disease without books is to sail an uncharted sea.' Study is also possible using virtual books. Tele-education, or education at a distance from the educator, is not a new concept. Textbooks, reference books and paper journals remain popular sources of information for health professionals, but they are being challenged, at least in terms of scope, cost and accessibility, by electronic resources. Web resources for neurologists are reviewed in Chapter 13. This chapter deals with the use of telemedicine for interactive educational meetings that incorporate distant participants (speakers, audience members, patient subjects). Lifelong learning is a requirement for neurologists, but due to the vast spectrum of neurological disease and relative local specialization, neurologists can become isolated educationally. Clinical isolation is also a risk, especially with respect to the rarer subspecialty interests of neurologists. Telecommunications offer some powerful solutions to these problems. There is an enormous range of communication technology available, including:

▶ paper/correspondence

▶ email

▶ audio/video recordings, broadcasts and downloads

▶ audio-conferencing
  – telephone
  – Internet telephony

▶ videoconferencing
  – integrated services digital network (ISDN) or asymmetric digital subscriber line (ADSL; broadband)
  – web-based

▶ broadcasting
  – satellite
  – television.

Many of these represent relatively low-technology approaches to tele-education that can be used in a wide variety of contexts and without substantial capital outlay.

Electronic correspondence

There are many possible ways of delivering an interactive meeting or education programme. Where live interaction is not necessary, email and Web-based teaching has been used successfully. Toyama and colleagues[1] described a regular educational nuclear medicine meeting using email correspondence. Interesting nuclear medicine images were selected by participants of the meeting and photographed using digital still cameras. The images and case descriptions were attached to email messages and sent to all members on a mailing list of participants. Any discussion points were added and replies were sent to all participants. Neuropathology and neuroradiology images could be disseminated and discussed in the same manner, and a simple email correspondence system would be ideal for clinical problem-solving exercises. Email meetings may be particularly suitable for international correspondence: time zones are irrelevant since replies do not have to be made in real time, and language barriers to communication can be reduced by automatic translation of email text. These electronic versions of the correspondence course have the advantage of rapid, cheap and easy distribution, with remote access and interactive correspondence. There is potential for real-time discussion using Web-based text or audio conferencing.

Audio conferencing

There appear to be few, if any, reports of the use of audio conferencing for neurology tele-education. The telephone is a simple, ubiquitous method for distance education.[2] Conferencing speakerphones are readily available for use with telephones. As an alternative to the telephone, Internet telephony is now of high quality and, importantly, can be free even for international connections, eg Skype.[3] Audio conferencing can be combined with printed material and/or emailed presentations, data and images.

Web-based videoconferencing using Microsoft NetMeeting software[4] transmits low-quality video in conjunction with audio. The low image resolution makes it unsuitable for the live transfer of the visual component of typical lectures. Its usefulness in medical education is not documented.

Electronic conferencing: video and audio streaming

There are many reports of the successful use of videoconferencing to deliver grand round and lecture material to geographically dispersed audience members. Web-based broadcasts use video and audio streaming. Streaming is a method of sending live video and audio information in a compressed digital format. The Internet tends to transfer data in a staccato fashion, but live audio and video need to appear seamless at the viewing end. Streaming is a complex process that involves creating, digitizing and transmitting data in a manner that appears live and smooth to the viewer/listener. For more information, see RealPlayer.[5] Such Web broadcasts can be accessed by multiple users, the only requirements being that they have Internet access and appropriate hardware and software for viewing and listening installed on their personal computers (PCs).[6,7]

For example, the Dartmouth-Hitchcock Medical School in the USA broadcasts live its neurology meeting, which occurs at midday local time. To hear and view the meeting, participants must have installed the RealPlayer software, which is available as a free download. I have attended this meeting from my home in the UK (17.00 local time) using a 300-kbit/s broadband connection. Audio transmits perfectly using this system. A live video of the slides has reduced resolution, even when viewed on a 38-cm computer monitor. Small print and figure details are significantly blurred, but slides usually convey sufficient information to illustrate the presentation. Questions can be asked of the presenter via email simply by clicking on an 'Ask the speaker a question' link in the presentation Web page. For the presenting institution, video streaming requires specific technical knowledge and software.[5] From the point of view of audience participants, this is a very simple and widely available interface to use. Video quality limits its usefulness for material that requires high-resolution images or projection on a large screen to multiple audience members. Its ready accessibility, whilst undoubtedly a great strength, limits its usefulness for presentation of patient material, where protecting patient confidentiality is paramount. The resolution and reliability of the connection depend critically on how the site is accessed, with a high-bandwidth local-area network (LAN) producing better results than a dial-up connection using a standard telephone line.

Attending a neurology lecture by video and audio streaming is simple. For example, the neurology grand rounds at the Dartmouth-Hitchcock Medical Centre are available via the Internet (Fig. 14.1).[8] Clearly, however, you will need to 'attend' at the correct time to have a successful connection to the live lecture. For the less well-organized, a series of pre-recorded neurology lectures is available for download from the website of the Massachusetts General Hospital.[9] These will provide an idea about the current capability of this technology.

Television and satellite communication

Television broadcasting, whether via a terrestrial or a satellite network, is expensive. If a large number of sites can be reached, then the unit costs may be affordable, at least in the short term. All of the work to date has concerned medical education across the entire spectrum, rather than being targeted specifically at neurology (which would probably make the economics even more difficult because the numbers are smaller).

For a small number of sites, satellite broadcasting may be too costly to be sustainable: the Mayo Clinic used a satellite video link between its three sites in the USA during the early 1990s[10] but ultimately changed to conventional (terrestrial) telecommunications. During the 1990s, the EuroTransMed Foundation for Continuing Medical Education broadcast interactive symposia on a range of medical topics, direct to hospitals, via television satellite.[11] The unit costs of delivering continuing professional development were estimated to be low,[12] and over a period of several years the operation expanded to encompass hospital sites in most of Western Europe. When the operation became

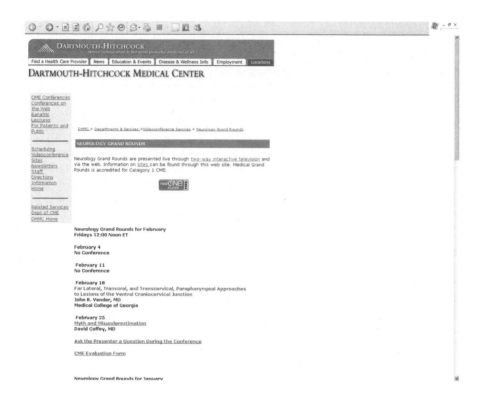

Fig. 14.1. Web page of neurology grand rounds at the Dartmouth-Hitchcock Medical Center.

financially unsustainable in 2001 and then ceased, it was broadcasting weekly to a network of over 250 hospitals in 27 countries in Western Europe.

The experience to date with television and satellite broadcasting for medical education suggests that the audience is simply not large enough to justify the costs. There are cheaper, if less glamorous, ways to deliver education to doctors.

Videoconference lectures using ISDN lines

In our institution, we have used ISDN connections for real-time videoconferences of neurology lectures and grand rounds. ISDN lines can carry more data than a telephone line (128 kbit/s versus 56 kbit/s), and we typically connect to remote centres using three ISDN lines, giving a bandwidth of 384 kbit/s. This gives a video quality that is adequate for video projection in a small (80 seats) lecture theatre (Fig. 14.2).

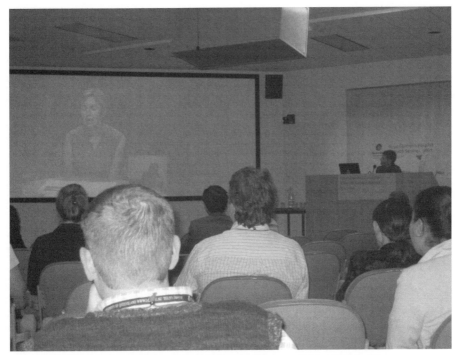

Fig. 14.2. Video lecture in progress, Royal Children's Hospital, Brisbane, Australia.

Presentation of remote patients

In Northern Ireland, patients of neurological interest can be presented at grand rounds, even if they live in distant parts of the country, by using the existing clinical teleneurology network. The patient can attend their local hospital and be presented by the teleneurology assistant over ISDN videoconferencing links to the central lecture theatre. The incoming image is presented on a monitor and also on a large screen using a data projector. History and physical examination can be conducted from the centre as in a normal videoconferenced clinic (see Chapter 4). Radiological images can be accessed from a Web server. It is important to inform the patient about the technology being used and to gain their consent for videoconferencing (Box 14.1).

Guest lectures

We have also used videoconferencing equipment to facilitate guest lecturers in delivering their talks without having to travel to our neurosciences meeting in Belfast. This saves lecturers a considerable amount of travel time and enables their expertise to

---

Box 14.1 Neurosciences Meeting: information for participants

The Neurosciences Meeting is a weekly meeting of medical professionals who are interested in diseases and disorders that affect the brain, spinal cord, nerves and muscles. The meeting is attended by doctors (neurologists, neurosurgeons, paediatric neurologists, neuroradiologists, neurophysiologists and neuropathologists), other healthcare professionals (eg physiotherapists, occupational therapists, nurses) and medical students.

Occasionally, some medical professionals may not be present at the meeting but are connected to the lecture theatre by a videoconferencing link. The videoconferencing connection is similar to a telephone connection, except that pictures as well as sound are transmitted. You will always be informed if someone is attending the meeting in this way, and you will be introduced to them so you are fully aware of everyone who is at the meeting.

Everything discussed at the Neurosciences Meeting is completely confidential. Videoconferencing allows a simple connection to another location – the sound and pictures are not recorded and are not broadcast in any way or put on the World Wide Web. If you require any clarification or have any questions about the meeting, please ask the doctors or nurses looking after you.

---

reach areas where it might not have done so otherwise. Most universities and teaching hospitals have videoconferencing equipment and, as video and audio transmission formats are standardized, equipment compatibility usually is not a major issue. One problem with such talks is ensuring that technical issues at the lecturer's site are sorted out. In our experience, most lecturers have limited experience with videoconferencing equipment, but technical staff members who are familiar with facilitating use of the technology are usually available. A first step in organizing a lecture is to contact the videoconferencing technical staff members at the institution of the guest speaker. Almost all practical aspects of the lecture can be organized by discussion with them, which therefore does not rely on the guest speakers involving themselves in technical issues.

The majority of technical problems can be anticipated or avoided by carrying out a test link between centres some days before the lecture (Table 14.1). This not only tests equipment compatibility, but also allows technical staff members to meet each other and the guest lecturer to become acquainted with the location and nature of the equipment.

Table 14.1. Methods of minimizing technical problems in videoconferences

- Test the link in advance of the meeting
  - if a new link is being used, then perform an initial test several days before the meeting.
  - commence the link at least 15 minutes before the meeting to re-check lighting, camera, sound/microphone and slide transmission.
- Ensure that remote participants know the location of conferencing equipment
- Ensure that technical support is available at all sites, as occasional technical problems are inevitable
- Obtain contact telephone/mobile numbers for speakers and technical staff

Remote meeting participation

The commonest reported use of videoconferencing for medical purposes is to allow remote audience participants to attend a central lecture.[13–15] This is particularly important for continuing medical education if practitioners are a long way from a regional centre or if healthcare providers are dispersed over a large area. There are increasing demands for continuing medical education from both practitioners and professional and statutory bodies, and the use of videoconferencing is an effective response to this in rural communities. It should be pointed out that when more than one distant site is connected to the centre, a multipoint videoconferencing bridge will be required.

Modifications required of videoconference presentations

Lecturers delivering a talk by videoconferencing need to be made aware of the limitations of the medium in order to optimize their presentations (Table 14.2). This process has many traps for the unwary. PowerPoint slides can be printed on paper and captured by video camera, but more commonly a device called a scan converter is used to convert the computer screen image to a video image, which is transmitted to the distant site. In general, scan converters are designed for converting static images, and therefore animated PowerPoint slides and embedded videos will not be transmitted. For this reason, the computer's mouse cursor is not an effective pointer for illustrating the slides. In addition, depending upon the quality of the scan converter, the resolution of the slide image and the legibility of the text may be diminished significantly; they will be reduced further if video projection on a large screen is required, because similar technology is used by data projectors.

The minimum legible text size varies according to several factors: technical factors concerning the quality of the scan converter; projection issues, such as the size of the projected image, ambient light and the quality of the video projector or monitor; and formatting issues, such as the slide colour scheme and the font used. Presenters therefore must keep their slides simple and use as large a font as possible with an uncomplicated background. Where high-resolution images and videos are important to the presentation, they should be sent in advance, either by email or on a CD or DVD by post.

Table 14.2. Limitations of videoconferencing for transmission of lecture slides

- Is the size of the text large enough for legibility?
- Is the contrast of the slide appropriate? (NB black lettering on a white background may offer too much contrast)
- Do graphs have too much detail?
- Are animated slides necessary?
- How will video be transmitted?
- Are the images and photographs of high enough resolution to reproduce properly?
- If there is a requirement for a pointer during the presentation, will it be visible at the remote sites?

Participant involvement in videoconference lectures

The key problem of videoconference lectures in comparison to traditional lectures is in the capacity for interaction of participants. A distant lecturer may be much more daunted by speaking to a television camera than to a live audience, especially if it is a novel experience. Their awareness of how their presentation is perceived is also reduced, as there is little immediate audience feedback through facial expression and body language. Audience members need to be comfortable with their local technology to contribute to discussions, and some participants may find this an additional barrier to being involved. On the other hand, animated multiple-voice discussions are stifled by the need for microphones and intelligible sound transmission. The chairperson in a videoconference meeting has a crucial role and must become skilled in involving the different sites and minimizing awareness of the technology. We find that everyone becomes increasingly relaxed about the lecture format as they become more familiar with it.

Evaluation

Evaluations of videoconference medical meetings have found them to be broadly acceptable for audiences. Lecturers tend to adapt quickly to using this technology.[15] In the evaluations of Sclater and colleagues[16] and Allen and colleagues,[17] lower satisfaction for audiences at the distant site relative to the central site were consistently observed. This relative dissatisfaction was related partly to slide legibility and technical problems with transmission, but satisfaction remained lower even when these factors were removed. Therefore, the live lecture remains the preferred format.

Conclusion

Our experience has been primarily with continuing postgraduate neurological education, where teaching usually takes the form of a lecture. This sort of programme plays to the strengths of communications technology – the knowledge of one expert speaker can be communicated at once to multiple listeners at multiple sites. Expert speakers have made themselves available because they do not have to bear the costs and time implications of travel. Didactic lecture formats lend themselves to videoconferencing with an initial broadcast followed by ordered discussion from speakers and questioners. ISDN videoconferencing therefore can improve the quality of lecture-based education by maximizing access to high-quality educators. As reliable higher-bandwidth Internet communication replaces ISDN, the ease of this process should increase and its costs decrease. Video streaming has arguably even greater potential to democratize access to the best of neurology education but, as in real-time clinical applications, intercontinental tele-education must contend with time differences. The lack of its widespread use, however, suggests that users are not yet overwhelmed by its quality and usefulness. Indeed, as the length of this chapter demonstrates, neurological tele-education is not yet a fully mature topic.

Further information

Kroodsma DE, Byers BE. Suggestions for Slides at Scientific Meetings. http://depts.washington.edu/bird2001/Slides.pdf. Accessed 11 February 2005.
Bellamy K, Mclean D. Using PowerPoint. *Journal of Audiovisual Media in Medicine* 2002; **25**: 162–164.
Communications Specialities, Inc. Six Common Misconceptions about Converting Computer to Video. www.commspecial.com/6misconc.htm. Accessed 11 February 2005.

References

1 Toyama H, Emoto Y, Ito K *et al*. Simple and low-cost tele-nuclear medicine conference system with the e-mail protocol. *Annals of Nuclear Medicine* 2001; **15**: 465–470.
2 Sheppard L, Mackintosh S. Technology in education: what is appropriate for rural and remote allied health professionals? *Australian Journal of Rural Health* 1998; **6**: 189–193.
3 Skype. www.skype.com. Accessed 11 February 2005.
4 NetMeeting. www.microsoft.com/windows/netmeeting/. Accessed 11 February 2005.
5 RealPlayer. www.real.com. Accessed 11 February 2005.
6 Rosser J, Herman B, Ehrenwerth C. An overview of videostreaming on the Internet and its application to surgical education. *Surgical Endoscopy* 2001; **15**: 624–629.
7 Gandsas A, McIntire K, Palli G, Park A. Live streaming video for medical education: a laboratory model. *Journal of Laparoendoscopic and Advanced Surgical Techniques Part A* 2002; **12**: 377–382.
8 Dartmouth-Hitchcock Medical Center. Neurology Grand Rounds. http://129.170.61.64/Neurology.htm. Accessed 11 February 2005.
9 Partners Neurology Grand Rounds. Online NeuroVideo Archives. http://neuro-www.mgh.harvard.edu/neurovideo. Accessed 11 February 2005.
10 Tangalos EG, McGee R, Bigbee AW. Use of the new media for medical education. *Journal of Telemedicine and Telecare* 1997; **3**: 40–47.
11 Geraghty JG, Young HL. Satellite-delivered continuing medical education in Europe. *Postgraduate Medical Journal* 1996; **72**: 218–220.
12 Young HL. Satellite-delivered medical education and training for central Europe: a TEMPUS project. Trans-European Mobility Programme for University Students. *Journal of Telemedicine and Telecare* 1996; **2**: 14–19.
13 McCrossin R. Successes and failures with grand rounds via videoconferencing at the Royal Children's Hospital in Brisbane. *Journal of Telemedicine and Telecare* 2001; **7** (suppl. 2): 25–28.
14 McCrossin R, Higgins N. Grand rounds at the Royal Children's Hospital in Brisbane. In Wootton R, Batch J, eds. *Telepediatrics: Telemedicine and Child Health*. London: Royal Society of Medicine Press, 2005; pp. 291–299.
15 Odell EW, Francis CA, Eaton KA *et al*. A study of videoconferencing for postgraduate continuing education in dentistry in the UK: the teachers' view. *European Journal of Dental Education* 2001; **5**: 113–119.
16 Sclater K, Alagiakrishnan K, Sclater A. An investigation of videoconferenced geriatric medicine grand rounds in Alberta. *Journal of Telemedicine and Telecare* 2004; **10**: 104–107.
17 Allen M, Sargeant J, MacDougall E, O'Brien B. Evaluation of videoconferenced grand rounds. *Journal of Telemedicine and Telecare* 2002; **8**: 210–216.

►15

Conclusion

Victor Patterson and Richard Wootton

Introduction

This book brings together for the first time the various strands that make up teleneurology. As editors, it is not our function to act as salespeople for teleneurology but rather to present a fair and unvarnished account of the field. To achieve this, we and our contributors have relied on the published literature, and we hope that in doing so we have not omitted any important work.

Techniques

The material in this book shows that teleneurology is possible using a range of techniques.

Telephone

The telephone is a much underrated medium for telemedicine in general. Its use in neurology provides a good example of how telemedicine is being used extensively in practice without any formal evidence of its safety or cost-effectiveness.

Email

Email use increases year on year, and the time cannot be far away when it will become the normal way for doctors to communicate with each other about patients. The National Health Service (NHS) in the UK seems determined to make this happen. When it does, then e-triage will seem a normal way of doing business, both in neurology and other specialties. For neurology in the developing world, the wider use of email will need more catalysts to realize its potential.

Videoconferencing

Videoconferencing can be made to work successfully, although it is still not as reliable in practice as it should be. The paediatric teleneurology work in Brisbane shows that videoconferencing can work successfully when coordinators provide technical and organizational assistance. This enables neurologists to practise neurology rather than worry about equipment. Trained teleneurology assistants at the remote end also make the process smoother for the hard-pressed neurologist.

Other forms of communication

Web chat and short message service (SMS) text messaging may well be used in neurology, but there is an absence of published literature regarding these forms of communication. This may change in the future.

Uses

Teleneurology is possible using a wide range of techniques. It has application across a broad spectrum of neurological disease.

Stroke

At present, the most rapid growth within teleneurology seems to be in the field of acute stroke care, where, for many people, telemedicine is the only solution to the specific problem of time-critical access to an effective medication. Its use in ill patients in this emergency situation proves that patients of all degrees of illness, however severe, can be assessed and managed by telemedicine.

Rehabilitation

The novel approaches to rehabilitation that telemedicine allows can be applied to many more people than at present. This ought to be a growth field for teleneurology, not only because it offers a potentially more efficient way of doing things, but also because potential beneficiaries are so very common.

Epilepsy

Epilepsy is a very common disease. People with this disorder are stigmatized and disadvantaged, especially if they live in rural areas, and most do not require the high-tech care of a comprehensive epilepsy centre. Neurological expertise makes a difference to these people, and telemedicine solutions do not require very sophisticated equipment. It is therefore quite extraordinary that so little epilepsy is managed by telemedicine. This ought to be a major growth area.

Neuroradiology

Neuroradiology is easily the most mature part of teleneurology and is embedded in everyday practice. This has happened because radiology is a huge part of medicine; it has used this critical mass to advance technologically, neuroradiology being included in the advance.

Neurophysiology

In contrast to neuroradiology, there are far fewer patients and specialists in neurophysiology, so the momentum for technological development has been less. In addition, although telemedicine brings advantages to the patients – reduced travel and improved access – there are no particular advantages to the doctors.

Success factors and barriers

Whether teleneurology is used or not depends on the doctors rather than the technology, because ultimately it requires doctors to recognize that teleneurology can benefit their patients. If the technology is appalling, enthusiastic doctors will still make it work. But even if the technology is top-notch, unconvinced doctors may not use it. This applies equally to doctors at both the specialist and remote ends of any telemedicine link.

A good relationship between the doctors involved in teleneurology is important, as are the coordinators, assistants and technical experts who all make the process smoother. Local champions are critical to telemedicine development, and without them the studies that form the basis for this book simply would not have taken place. They have the lack of arrogance to realize that others can improve the care of their patients and possess the ability to make the organizational changes that allow telemedicine to prosper. They are the largely unsung heroes of teleneurology.

Sceptical doctors are more likely to change if there is some evidence of cost benefit,[1] and this is where the proponents of teleneurology can help, by providing some evidence for their endeavours. Their enthusiasm will then become evidence-based enthusiasm. Some criticism has been made about the lack of evidence for telemedicine in general,[2,3] but in the front-line clinical areas that teleneurology is seeking to improve, randomized controlled trials are difficult to do, sometimes because of ethical concerns and sometimes because the benefits, like that of the parachute,[4] are so blindingly obvious (Fig. 15.1).

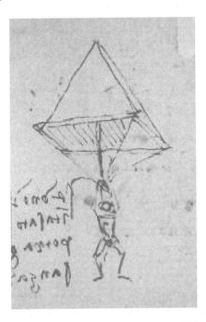

Fig. 15.1. The benefits of the parachute were recognized at least 500 years ago. And yet, to date, there has been no randomized controlled trial ...

The future

It is neither possible nor desirable to do all neurology by telemedicine. However, it is clear that telemedicine can be used in ways that bring benefits to neurological patients, their healthcare providers and even their neurologists. These benefits extend from acute neurology to community rehabilitation, and from patients in the next village to those on distant continents. The tools range from the latest expensive videoconferencing equipment to the humble email message sent via a dial-up connection. The latter can be used almost anywhere and has the potential to help more people in more countries than any other form of teleneurology.

Teleneurology is a microcosm of telemedicine as a whole. It is a cottage industry, heavily dependent on 'people factors' for success. Nonetheless, as this book shows, teleneurology can be used successfully by neurologists and can help a number of their patients. In global terms, the numbers of neurologists using telemedicine, and of patients benefiting from it, are still small. If both of these numbers increase, then this book will have succeeded in its aim.

References

1   McCrossin R. Managing risk in telemedicine. *Journal of Telemedicine and Telecare* 2003; **9** (suppl. 2): 36–39.
2   Hailey D, Ohinmaa A, Roine R. Study quality and evidence of benefit in recent assessments of telemedicine. *Journal of Telemedicine and Telecare* 2004; **10**: 318–324.
3   Hailey D, Roine R, Ohinmaa A. Systematic review of evidence for the benefits of telemedicine. *Journal of Telemedicine and Telecare* 2002; **8** (suppl. 1): 1–30.
4   Smith GCS, Pell JP. Parachute use to prevent death and major trauma related to gravitational challenge: systematic review of randomised controlled trials. *British Medical Journal* 2005; **327**: 1459–1461.

▶ Index

Page numbers in *italics* refer to information in figures or tables